# HYPNOTISM

Fundamental Principles and Practice for Beginners

(A Hypnotherapists Guide to Hypnotising in Person and Online)

**Junie Farthing**

Published by Andrew Zen

**Junie Farthing**

All Rights Reserved

*Hypnotism: Fundamental Principles and Practice for Beginners (A Hypnotherapists Guide to Hypnotising in Person and Online)*

ISBN 978-1-77485-238-5

All rights reserved. No part of this guide may be reproduced in any form without permission in writing from the publisher except in the case of brief quotations embodied in critical articles or reviews.

Legal & Disclaimer

The information contained in this book is not designed to replace or take the place of any form of medicine or professional medical advice. The information in this book has been provided for educational and entertainment purposes only.

The information contained in this book has been compiled from sources deemed reliable, and it is accurate to the best of the Author's knowledge; however, the Author cannot guarantee its accuracy and validity and cannot be held liable for any errors or omissions. Changes are periodically made to this book. You must consult your doctor or get professional medical advice before using any of the suggested remedies, techniques, or information in this book.

Upon using the information contained in this book, you agree to hold harmless the Author from and against any damages, costs, and expenses, including any legal fees potentially resulting from the application of any of the information provided by this guide. This disclaimer applies to any damages or injury caused by the use and application, whether directly or indirectly, of any advice or information presented, whether for breach of contract, tort, negligence, personal injury, criminal intent, or under any other cause of action.

You agree to accept all risks of using the information presented inside this book. You need to consult a professional medical practitioner in order to ensure you are both able and healthy enough to participate in this program.

# Table of Contents

INTRODUCTION .................................................................. 1

CHAPTER 1: HYPNOSIS AND MIND CONTROL .................... 4

CHAPTER 2: FUNDAMENTALS OF HYPNOSIS..................... 22

CHAPTER 3: SELF HYPNOSIS AS A METHOD TO POSITIVE CHANGE ........................................................................... 37

CHAPTER 4: A SHORT BACKGROUND OF HYPNOSIS......... 42

CHAPTER 5: WHAT DOES IT MEAN?................................. 47

CHAPTER 6: ARE YOU CONNECTED? ................................ 53

CHAPTER 7: WHAT IS HYPNOSIS? .................................... 64

CHAPTER 8: REGRESSION METHODS ............................... 81

CHAPTER 9: THE MODEL................................................... 89

CHAPTER 10: UNDERSTANDING HYPNOSIS...................... 92

CHAPTER 11: HYPNOSIS MP3S - A TECHNOLOGY ADVANTAGE...................................................................... 97

CHAPTER 12: HOW TO BECOME A HYPNOTIST .............. 115

CHAPTER 13: THE FEAR OF THE DARK THINKING ........... 126

CHAPTER 14: CLASSICAL FORMS OF SUGGESTIVE INFLUENCE ..................................................................... 135

CHAPTER 15: UNDERSTANDING HYPNOSIS.................... 144

CHAPTER 16: THE REASONS NLP IS WORKING FOR SELP-HELP? ............................................................................. 155

**CHAPTER 17: REDEFINING THE MIND ............................ 165**

**CHAPTER 18: WHAT HYPNOSIS CAN AND CAN'T DO ...... 172**

**CONCLUSION ................................................................. 184**

## Introduction

There could be a myriad of reasons for you to want to start your own business.

Maybe, you're looking for economic rewards, or perhaps the freedom to manage your own company with your personal choices. Perhaps, you like the challenge of creating your own business's success (financial and not). Perhaps you long for the chance to showcase your individual talents and capabilities.

Naturally, with potential rewards, comes some risk. It is possible to risk your job or your financial situation and even put the security of your family at risk. While nothing in life is without risk, you'd surely want to minimize your risk to the maximum extent feasible.

This guidebook will assist you reduce your risk and maximize your reward by accessing the most powerful source that you have the sub-conscious mind, and its incredible power!

Whatever the reason you're looking to start your own business this ebook will assist you to dig into your unconscious to find your own uniqueness and then to create and manage your own business venture built around your specific talents.

The method is based on six tools made up of a mixture of

6. Clear, dependable and well-established business concepts. (.to follow what is in line with business sense)

7. The incredible power of the hypnosis process. (to help you focus, or awaken your unique business skills)

8. The transformative capabilities that are unleashed by subliminals embedded. (to 'embed' your success qualities)

The six tools for business that are easy to use give you a great beginning point to become an entrepreneur who is successful. The guideline is a step-by-step procedure that you can use in any venture, regardless of whether you want to use it within or outside of a company, and whether you'd like to become an IN-TREPRENEUR, and/or an E-TREPRENEUR.

# Chapter 1: Hypnosis and Mind Control

Let's begin with an explanation of what hypnosis actually is. Hypnosis is a method of manipulating the mind which involves not only the direct participation of the individual being in hypnosis, but also the direction of the entire process. As we will see in chapter on stage hypnosis, and other chapters in the book, hypnosis does independent of any specific charisma or talent on the part of the person who is hypnotized. The hypnotist is an instructor, working in conjunction with the person in a state of trance and is the one driving the process. Hypnosis, when distilled into basic terms, is a kind of induced trance which is distinct from the natural sleep. In hypnosis, a person is directed to focus entirely on one specific thing such as emotion, problem, or idea without regard to other aspects of the awake world. This means that the subject is focused on the one thought or thing that is at the focus that is hypnotized. Thus the mental and physical capacities of the person work in relation to this particular idea throughout the time they are in the influence of hypnosis. In essence, when hypnosis is in effect it is the case that the concentration of the subject increases, while other aspects of their mind become diminished. It's a great way to eliminate distractions.

There are typically two people who are involved in a hypnosis session that is the hypnotist as well as the person who is being at the receiving end of hypnosis. The role of a person who is hypnotized in a hypnosis session is to lead the patient to a state of hypnosis sleep, and also to guide them in their perception of things and thoughts that are that are in their mind. The hypnotist can guide the subject through all senses including touch, smell and. Everything the subject smells, perceives or hears is one of the methods used by the hypnotist's effort to direct the subject towards an idea or object. Hypnosis for self (or autohypnosis) is also a type of hypnosis that is only for the person who is. The subject has to direct their self-hypnosis to the object or concept of interest or focus. This is the type of hypnotism more in depth later in the book.

Hypnotism is basically granting an access point to the subconscious mind and subconscious mind. You might be wondering what the subconscious mind and what is important to are able to access it. The conscious mind acts as the storage space of all that we've observed, felt, or experienced during our lives. Consider the skill you have to master, such as driving in a car. In the first few times you are driving a car the car, you'll be focused exclusively on driving and not be able on the conversations happening within the car. It's because your mind isn't able to retain the ability. After a while of training, driving will become easily to you. What's the reason? Because the knowledge you've gained through your driving experience will be stored in your mind's subconscious. This means that your subconscious is now driving the car.

The information stored in your brain's subconscious to steer, while your conscious mind is focused on the conversations in the car. It is the subconscious mind that is is responsible for the emotions and emotions that you experience whenever you face any new circumstance. For instance, if you were to take part in an audition The fear and anxiety you feel comes due to your subconscious mind which has stored your feelings and linked it to things that might make you feel embarrassed. you. The subconscious mind is the one that controls the involuntary movements of our bodies like breathing. It is essentially in charge from the time we are introduced into this world until the moment that we leave it.

The conscious mind is on the other hand is the one the brain responsible for all reasoning and reasoning that we employ. The conscious mind makes up just 10-12% of our cognitive capacity. The rest can be attributed to our unconscious and subconscious mind. It is your conscious brain that that you employ to solve challenges, come up with solutions, and use on a regular basis. It houses the working memory, the memory we require for functioning on a regular basis. It is the control for our logical, analytical capabilities and bodily actions.

We've now talked about the differentiators between our unconscious, our subconscious and conscious minds it is important to know that hypnotism doesn't only get your subconscious mind to listen. It's a state of mid-level consciousness, in which your mind is more receptive to suggestions. Two theories exist regarding what happens when hypnosis is achieved. One theory, called"the altered state hypothesis states that when someone is in a state of hypnosis, a trance begins to develop. The theory suggests that the trance state is your unconscious. A second hypothesis (non-state) states that when someone is hypnotized the role they imagine for themselves is playing. It asserts that it's more of an active mental state, where the person believes that they have all the desirable traits however reality can challenge the assumption.

## The altered state theory of Hypnosis

The theory of altered state hypnosis isn't the current concept of what takes place during the state of hypnosis "state" and comes originally, from mesmerism. Mesmerism's basic premise was that the hypnotist positioned the subject in an altered state which was distinct from conscious, allowing the subject to be more susceptible to suggestions. A vast amount of research on the effects in hypnosis proved that this theory is not valid, which has led to a better understanding, especially in relation to hypnotherapy's effectiveness for many who suffer from depressive symptoms, PTSD as well as stress.

## The non-state theory of the hypnosis

This is the contemporary concept of the practice of hypnosis. In this way the mind state isn't altered so much as the mind is opened by an invitation and encouragement by the practitioner. This opens up more openness to the person being studied. In allowing for a greater imagination, the suggestion is processed differently, whether through non-verbal or verbal directions. This allows the subject to be more apt to receive useful information that can trigger an alteration in the perspective. This can be the basis to resolving existing issues as demonstrated through the study on returning combat veteran Gary earlier in the book. Professor. Gerling, by directing Gary to examine the traumatizing events he had experienced in the field as an observer, and then to engage in the battle to face his past self, helped him to begin seeing these events with greater confidence. In this manner, Gary was able to deal with his PTSD better and live an unfettered life free of the negative effects of PTSD.

The difference between the two theories marks an dividing line between the previous interpretations of hypnosis and its functions as well as the more modern interpretation. While the earlier understanding might be more in need of further advancement, the research of early hypnosis specialists like James Braid are of foundational importance for the contemporary understanding of the processes. Similar to those theories developed by Freud and his colleagues, which are no longer crucial to the clinical practice of psychiatry the way they were in the past the altered state theory was still an effective framework to further develop. In this moment, it's vital that I clarify some words that are used throughout the book. Terms like "trance" are a good example. They are used to provide readers with access. It's a word that is widely used to describe how the mind responds to the hypnosis. This isn't to suggest, however, that nothing about the mind changes. It's the same mind, made up from the identical functions and material. It is simply opened to the working with the hypnotic suggestion to allow for the perception of perspective to be guided towards the direction of change.

Hypnotherapy benefits and benefits of it

As we've mentioned earlier that hypnosis is commonly employed as a method of therapy. It is often employed as a method of relaxation. Hypnotherapy as the medical practice is referred to as, is often used to induce a state calm. It is also widely employed to treat emotional, psychological as well as physical issues. The disorders treated with hypnotherapy range from stress to obsessional-compulsive disorder. The degree that hypnotherapy can be effective depends on the willingness of an person to be hypnotized and the severity that the condition is. If someone is forcefully forced to attend the hypnosis sessions the session is likely to be unsuccessful since their mind won't be able to cooperate with the practitioner. Some people, when they have the increasing frequency of sessions, the mind may eventually be able to cooperate and be controlled by the person who is hypnotizing. Some people aren't responsive to hypnosis due to the inability to build trust.

We've covered a few ways that hypnosis and hypnotherapy has been developed over the years to aid in overcoming psychological difficulties. There are also many practical advantages associated with its use, and we'll examine.

Stress relief

Hypnotherapy can be beneficial in reducing stress levels. We are all overwhelmed by our daily lives. It is now recognized that stress can affect our physical health, so individuals are turning to alternate treatments such as hypnotherapy to help. Hypnotherapy is just one of the many methods to help reduce the negative effects that stress can have on well-being. By assisting your mind and body to rest, it may offer more than just a means of relaxing, but as well (with the help of a practitioner) aid you in dealing more effectively with stress.

Self-hypnosis will be discussed more in the near future however guided imagery as well as visualization are the basis of this and, in regards to stress-relief this self-hypnosis aspect could be a pleasant part of a hectic day.

Depression and anxiety

Patients suffering with depression and anxiety often encounter the situation that prescription medication does not suffice to relieve the symptoms. Many of them turn to the practice of hypnotherapy. Hypnotherapy can help people tackle the causes of depression and get rid of them one by one. Regular treatment with hypnotherapy could result in a significant reduction in the symptoms and assist sufferers to live more fulfilled lives.

A lot of sufferers of cancer and PTSD sufferers might be struggling with depression and anxiety and, with more doctors using complementary treatments as an alternative to traditional methods and hypnotherapy has helped those who are suffering unnecessarily.

Recovery from addiction

Many people are afflicted with addictions because of their environment as well as their genetic predisposition. Certain people are more vulnerable to the temptation of drugs, gambling and alcohol, in addition to cravings for food and sexual. There are many hypnotherapy strategies employed that are beneficial for those trying to conquer addiction. The methods help addicts to control their thoughts to overcome addiction and lead life in a healthy, full way. While it is not recommended as a solution to the scourge of addiction, it has been proven to be effective in certain instances. The use of it as a complement to treatment for addicts in need of treatment is growing in popularity within the therapy community.

Addicts are usually confronted by negative self-image issues which 12 Step programs do not deal with. Indeed, organizations such as AA that force addicts to be in front of the group and announce their addiction as an unchangeable life-style, could cause the merry-go-round experience experienced among addicts. By focusing on the neural pathways in the brain, a highly skilled professional can assist patients in getting off the merry go-round. They can help their patients make fundamental shifts in their self-perception and moving toward a more positive image of themselves towards positive self-image they are helping several addicts and helping them free from the trap of addiction.

## Pain relief

Migraines and arthritis are two conditions which cause lots of discomfort. Painkillers are the primary treatment for these diseases. But, if drugs don't work it is possible to try hypnotherapy as an alternative. Hypnotherapy, which has the ability to convince your brain that the pain can be controlled can be a powerful method to lessen the pain in certain instances.

Particularly relevant to women is the impact of hypnosis in the process of birth. Psychoprophylactic methods are used to doctors talk about the impending birth with women who are pregnant, along with the use of hypnosis. The most effective method is to protect minds from trauma of having a baby. Women who self-hypnotize during labor also say that their pain is lessened but not completely eliminated.

## Relaxation

Relaxation is a method to improve the health of the mind as well as the body. It is important for us to relax and concentrate. A person who is calm and calm generally aren't irritable or upset quickly. Relaxed people are also less likely to suffer from various lifestyle ailments like heart attacks, strokes and other cardiovascular ailments. It is possible to attain the state of calm through hypnosis and utilize self-hypnosis as a way to maintain your peace when under stress or stress. Hypnosis may have long-lasting positive effects and can greatly improve overall well-being, for instance.

Weight loss

Hypnotherapy can be employed as part to a loss plan. It isn't so simple as simply implementing an eating plan. Certain people are overweight because they eat too much due to mental illness that causes them to consume food. Other people are overweight due to glandular issues and the genetics of heredity. Hypnotherapy is a great way to help people put their weight issues into the right perspective and cope with them better. Many people who are on the weight loss plan have issues with self-esteem which can be cured or even eliminated through the use of hypnotherapy. Like with addiction, changing the foundational attitudes about one's self-image are crucial to help them shed excess weight. When weight loss was accomplished in order to protect the self against the outside world and the world, there may be deeper issues involved (sexual abuse is just one) that is able to be discovered and resolved by therapy with hypnotherapy.

Sleep disorders

Sleep disorders can range in severity from sleeplessness to nightmares. These conditions affect hundreds of people. They causes many to have insomnia for long periods of time. Sleep deprivation is an unintentional stressor for the body. The body's clock gets confused and this could cause serious harm to the mechanisms that allow the body to function, causing health problems. People gain weight if they do not sleep regularly, while others shed significant weight. There are even cases of various illnesses due to this absence of sleep. Other medications and sleeping pills can have negative impacts on the body. Sleeping problems are usually psychological which is why they require some amount of psychotherapy alongside physical treatment. Hypnosis is a factor in the treatment of sleep disorders because it helps patients achieve an environment where their minds are not in a high-activity state. This is particularly beneficial for those suffering from sleep disturbance due to PTSD.

Changes in behavior

Hypnosis is a method to induce behavior changes (as is the case for those who suffer from trouble with addiction). People who struggle with anger management may benefit from hypnosis as an technique to control their urges. Hypnosis allows people to control their lives, and also to lessen the negative effects of violent eruptions that may be caused by an inability to manage anger abilities.

Recall memories that were buried

Repressed memories are the result of the abuse we endured as an infant. To safeguard our minds from these memories they are buried in our sub-conscious. While there is much debate regarding this theory that we can bury our memories, there is enough evidence to suggest that humans are capable of removing information from the conscious mind in order to guard against emotional trauma that comes with past traumas. (See the section regarding Regression therapy).

Hypnotherapy is a method to bring these memories back to better recognize the pain we've suffered and the impact it had on our lives as we grow older. It is also a method to relive joyful memories that could have been lost by an accident or fall or a fall, as well as life abilities, skills, and motor abilities that are lost due because of a Traumatic Brain Injury (TBI).

Apart from these advantages In addition, hypnotherapy lets people live happier lives by enhancing their general attitude. After a person has a few hypnosis sessions, they will be more relaxed and calm. The relaxed state of mind is what makes them attractive to hang around with. Hypnosis can also help them be in a state of mind that is clear which allows them to be more imaginative and effective in their work lives, and. Hypnotherapy is commonly employed as a means to success. Instead of guiding people directly towards success, it guides them the steps they need to take to get there. If lack of self-confidence is the sole factor that prevents someone from getting to where they want to be and hypnotherapy is the solution, it can aid them in regaining their confidence and allow them to become more in charge over their life and lead life more completely.

## Chapter 2: Fundamentals of Hypnosis

It is likely that you've had a trance experience in the realm of fantasy. Typically, the story is as follows the mentalist whispers to a person who is a trusted subject to induce them into the state of trance. The subject is then hypnotized and follows every instruction of the person who is hypnotizing them. If you're a serious film buff Svengali's name might bring to mind. The George du Maurier-written gothic horror novel Trillby The evil villain Svengali employs hypnosis in order to transform the main character the young tone-deaf English girl to become a performer. She is kept in a state of hypnosis in which he is able to manipulate and exploit her.

It's terrifying to think that there are people who are skilled in mind control, who can use just a few words and turn others into their minds to be their slaves, isn't it? Perhaps you're contemplating, "Cool!

What can I do to master that technique?" You may also be one of those doubtful and believe that the possibility of hypnosis.

The use of hypnosis actually exists. In actual fact, it's widely accepted and acknowledged within the field of health care as a valid medical procedure. It's a good thing, unlike other kinds of procedures that require an expert in the field to carry out the procedure, hypnosis can be used by anyone. That is what you'll learn. Before I go into the different methods of hypnosis and how you can apply them to your own and others, we'll start by introducing the basics and debunk the technique of hypnosis.

The art of separating Fact from Fiction

Let me be clear in real life: the process of hypnosis does not look as dramatic as the often over-dramatized portrayals in the world of fake believe. Therefore, let's look at some of the myths that are commonly attributed to it and clear off the table. Here are the most important facts about hypnosis:

MyTH: Hypnosis is black magic

Truth: There is no hocus-pocus about the practice. Hypnosis has been used successfully in the field of medicine from the 50s. While trance states that resemble being hypnotized have been observed and utilized by shamans as well as faith healers in the rituals of various cultures across the globe there is a scientific basis for this. I will discuss more in Chapter 2.

Myth A skilled hypnotist will make anyone feel controlled in their mind.

The truth is that if you're contemplating learning to hypnotize in order to be able to control and influence the minds of others people, you'll be disappointed. However should you be hesitant about being hypnotized then let me assure you that there is nothing to worry about. We've already proven that hypnosis in the media is erroneous and exaggerated. So, who are the is the stage performers are hypnotists? I'm talking about those who choose an uninvolved member of the audience, place them under hypnosis and let them whine and waddle like a duck to make fun of them. However, stage hypnotists are mostly as entertainers first, just like illusionists. The actors they bring on stage aren't individuals who are not really strangers in any way and are, in reality, either participants in the act, or are highly adept at hypnotizing (more about the subject in chapter 5). This is the most crucial aspect of the art of hypnosis: no person can be hypnotized against wishes.

Myth: With hypnosis other treatments and medications can be obliterated

Fact: The practice of hypnotherapy -- one form of psychotherapy that employs the use of hypnosis in the process has been proved to be a successful treatment for many ailments that range from allergies and chronic pain to depression and anxiety, even poor behaviors or low self-esteem. In certain situations, particularly when it comes to emotional-based disorders it's even suggested as the first option for treatment. However, it has its limitations and is not able to replace all other treatments. Since hypnosis focuses on the mind, it's ideal for conditions that are rooted in the mind, and have no physical basis. Disorders like anxiety and depression, as well as chronic stress, paranoia and addiction can greatly benefit from the practice of hypnotherapy. In most instances it can be beneficial as a complement to any treatment program. It is not possible to hypnotize the pain of a broken bone or tumor However, you can utilize methods of hypnosis to reduce the pain and get mentally ready for surgery.

Myth: Hypnosis can be dangerous since it can play with your brain.

A FACT: Caution must be taken when you plan to utilize hypnosis in order to assist those suffering from serious mental disorders. In these cases a certified professional hypnotherapist is recommended. Other than that simple hypnosis is completely secure.

Myth: Hypnosis is an enlightenment state

The brainwaves recorded in both meditation and hypnosis is the same, they are completely different, and have distinct goals. The purpose for meditation is entering into an altered state of mind and concentrate on your own inner thoughts, and focus on yourself. The purpose of hypnosis would be to enter the same state of mind and then get suggestions in order to alter your thought, behaviour or habit.

MyTH: Hypnosis is similar to sleep.

Fact: This is a myth that has been prevalent for centuries due to the term "hypnosis" that comes in the Greek word meaning sleep, the word hypnos. While you sleep, your brain is able to drift off and, unless you are disturbed you have no awareness of the world around you. From one's face, the effects of hypnosis may appear like sleep, as the person who is hypnotized might appear relaxed in their sleep, even with their eyes shut. But, the person is in fact alert and is able to perceive the happenings within their environment.

Myth: Being hypnotized is simply a state of deep relaxation

The truth is that while it's simpler for someone to be hypnotized at a level of calm and a relaxed state, it's not required. As you'll discover later , hypnosis is able to be achieved in any state. However, you should be hypnotized only when you're relaxed for a relaxing experience.

Myth It is possible to be hypnotized and not even conscious of it

Fact: Of the many myths about the hypnosis process, this one may have a tiny bit of truth. You might be shocked to learn that hypnosis actually is more commonplace in life than you thought. Keep on...you might be thinking, isn't this in contradiction to what I said earlier about the inability to utilize hypnosis for controlling your thoughts? But, no, it's not. which brings me to my next thing...

You're being In a state of Hypnosis Right Now!

If I said you could be hypnotized, without even realizing it, I meant that we have every one of us been in a kind of situation in which we were unaware of amazing messages and suggestions that are being fed into our brains. The messages are a blue print that affects how we think about, act, and the decisions we make.

Actually, our first experience with hypnosis comes through our guardianship and parents figures. Take a look at all the things you were constantly told as a young person as to what you should or should not do according to your parents. Then, think about certain behaviors of beliefs, values, and beliefs that you've cultivated throughout your early years, which your parents and moms taught you, and which can still influence your thinking in certain ways. The mind of a child is exposed to both visual and verbal information it is exposed to in a variety of ways. Therefore, the knowledge and concepts that were ingrained in us in our early years were deeply embedded in our minds that can be difficult to remove in adulthood. The reason for this is our brains being able to create mental connections.

In simple terms If we experience something that happens in our lives, the brain will record the event and formulate something of reaction. When we come across a similar scenario, all of the physical and emotional responses that we have associated with the memory are dredged into the sand. To provide one example of this, ask you to look at the first thoughts that pop to your mind when I suggest you think of the rose. Think about the rose's stunning hue, its softness the petals offer, the fragrance and its thorny stem what emotions do those images evoke in you? Perhaps you remember a wonderful moment, or perhaps someone gifted to you a beautiful bouquet of flowers on Valentine's Day. You might consider someone who is a fan of scents of florals. The scent, smell and feel of a rose can bring the sensation of feeling loved loved. It means that you're in positive associations with the rose.

However, mental associations can also be negative. Referring to the rose illustration Let me share an example that is often mentioned to illustrate how physical ailments can begin within the mind. There was a lady who was so allergic to roses. Whenever she was in proximity to the flowers, itching were seen across her entire skin. Naturally, doctors concluded that she was allergic to the chemical constituents of the flowers. One day, when she was visiting a close friend and walked into the room and saw an arrangement of roses in a vase. Likely, she experienced an allergy reaction...only to discover that the flowers were made of plastic. To find the cause of the issue she sought out an hypnotherapist who placed her in a trance and helped her remember the incidents that led to getting the allergy. Then it was realized that her aversion to roses resulted from a stifled childhood memory. It turned out that while this girl was a kid and reached to a vase with roses that she was not supposed to play with, which caused it to drop from the shelf. The woman was severely punished for her mistake and the memory stayed with her, creating a negative psychological image of roses. If unchecked the negative mental images are likely to manifest into the development of addiction, bad habits or even physical ailments.

You might be thinking that if a child's brain can be easily programmed surely an adult who can think independently would be able to tell what they are thinking about being affected. Then, we'd be able to resist considering that, as I stated previously, no one can be controlled by their own will, isn't it? Although it's true that nobody can provide thoughts or suggestions to cause you to think and behave in a particular way however, they are certainly able to influence your thinking. If their influence is enough, you could be compelled by the influence to follow your own accord in accordance with what others want you to act. There is no need to look far to find the perfect example for this kind of the hypnosis. They're everywhere. They appear on TV with your most loved programs, you hear them on the radio in between your favourite songs, and while you read an online news article you will see them in the corner, calling for you to click. These are advertisements. Adverts are, in fact, the most effective at hypnotizing!

There's a reason an individual brand will pop out of your head every time you think of something. Advertisers are skilled at creating hypnotic imagery and scripts to penetrate the corners of our minds , gradually infusing their brand's name, slogan, and images in our minds. While it's technically possible to be aware that you're being hypnotized, and you can fight it, the reality is that staying alert requires a large quantity of energy. As I've mentioned previously, nobody is able to use hypnosis to alter the will of an individual. Imagine a restaurant to eat, an expensive premium smartphone, an efficient skincare product or an elegant bag; what brand is immediately in your mind? What does that mean? that you'd really want to purchase that products? It's not unless you truly would like to, surely? The point I'm trying highlight is that you may be tricked into thinking and thinking something. However, in the end it's your responsibility to make a decision based on that information. So, there is absolutely nothing to worry about when it comes to the process of hypnosis. If you are able to break free from a convincing selling pitch, you could be free of being hypnotized at any time.

Then, what exactly is Hypnosis?

If you've learned that the difference between hypnosis and an untruth used by swindlers and that there is no magic involved, your curiosity is likely to be piqued and you're eager to learn the mechanism behind it do you not? You might be asking how hypnosis works? Numerous studies have been conducted to comprehend the process that makes hypnosis feasible. As of now, researchers have not succeeded in their quest to find the solution. There are a variety of theories, some of which contradict other theories. I won't discuss the details of these theories since they will only serve to confuse you more.

We've established the things that hypnosis does not. Therefore, all you have to know is that hypnosis can be an instrument that you can use to aid your self and others in numerous ways by harnessing the power of your mind. The effectiveness of this technique is dependent on two important elements:

1.) Ability of the to hypnotize.

2.) The level of cooperation displayed by the person who is being hypnotized.

Why are you hypnotized?

After I've (hopefully) put the mind in a calm state, I've one final thing to inform you, and that's the reason you should take a course in the art of hypnosis. It is a simple fact that this extremely powerful tool is able to enhance your life in numerous ways. By using hypnosis, it is possible to:

o Improve general health, and overall well-being. We should not forget that hypnosis is as a remedy for certain ailments, particularly in connection to the brain. Maybe you have a habit that's harmful to your overall health that you must get rid of or perhaps you aren't able to adhere to a diet plan for weight loss for long enough. Are you struggling with a kind of anxiety or chronic discomfort? Hypnosis may help you get there.

o Overcome barriers. When used correctly, hypnosis can be extremely effective to help you overcome the fear of speaking in public or nightmares. You can also overcome unfounded fears that are keeping you from doing the thing you love. It is also a great way to prepare yourself for stressful and frightening situations, like child birth, surgery, and even tattoos!

• Improve your ability. It could be more concentration or increasing your golf skills or controlling your time more effectively using hypnosis, it allows you to increase your mental abilities.

## Chapter 3: Self Hypnosis As A Method To Positive Change

Self-hypnosis is a method that has many advantages that include physical, emotional benefits, as well as mental wellbeing. Self-hypnosis is completely secure, relaxing and stimulating.

Self-hypnosis is a method of use to do other than just relaxing. Many people are unaware of the benefits of self-hypnosis. Self-hypnosis can be used to connect with the subconscious mind and change the ways we think and act.

Self-hypnosis is a method to transform many aspects of your life. The use of self-hypnosis is to eliminate negative emotions associated from bad memories. It is possible to use self-hypnosis to get rid of negative beliefs and to create new ones. You could also utilize self-hypnosis to accomplish objectives!

To reap the maximum benefits from self-hypnosis, it is important to understand the reasons you're making use of it. Self-hypnosis without prior intent will be a sign that what you will gain from it is just relaxing. Create a goal for self-hypnosis! Self-hypnosis has been proven to provide physical and mental revitalization and can aid in maintaining an optimistic mindset. Hypnosis can help individuals to concentrate on a variety of issues, and boost self-esteem.

Self-hypnosis used to improve self-esteem is becoming increasingly popular for a lot of individuals. The variety of hypnosis methods and methods of self-hypnosis for getting the mind into a state of trance, as well as self-hypnosis publications or manuals are becoming increasingly popular. But the most effective method to master the art of successful self-hypnosis is to learn directly from a trained and skilled hypnotherapist.

In essence, self-hypnosis can be taught to improve self-esteem regardless of the stage the individual can attain from a trance that is light or deep relaxation. Hypnosis to effect positive change is about putting yourself in the mindset of a different person so that you can expand the possibilities and discover innovative ways to tackle problems. Hypnosis for self-hypnosis is only restricted by your imagination.

To make a positive impact one must:

Make a goal and record the goal in writing. The self-hypnosis goal must be clear and concise. When you write down your statement of intention, you cement your idea of what you would like to accomplish in your mind . It also gives your mind something that it has to focus on.

The aim should be your own as well as achievable, positive and should be stated in the present sentence. Make a written declaration that only contains the things you wish to achieve and must not be focused in any way, on things you do not want to be experiencing anymore. Examples of positive phrases would be "I attain my ideal weight effortlessly" instead of "I have lost weight". The mind is a visual organ and when you concentrate on not being overweight, your mind makes up a mental picture of you being overweight.

You might, for instance, need hypnosis to help you improve yourself and to have a high self-esteem. The goals could include:
"I am content to always keep my head up high and be happy.'

One can always experiment with the words that are used to describe the purpose to ensure that the phrase truly means something to you. If you follow this advice, you will ensure that the sole images that your mind makes are positive. When you self-hypnotize, you recall these images it is telling the subconscious to aid you construct them.

To practice, you can take a look at the statement you written and begin to become aware of the images you're seeing in your head. The images you see will be larger as well as more vibrant and emotional. Change the mental picture until it's exactly as you want it to be in real life. If you can imagine that the words are true, then feel how you will feel if these statements were true now and right now. Continue to change it until you feel great. The written words and mental images, along with positive feelings are the basis for successful self-hypnosis.

## Chapter 4: A Short Background of Hypnosis

Hypnotism was born out of mesmerism as a method is the practice of using and having "animal-magnetism" along with the idea being a "magnetic liquid" was first discovered by an German doctor named Franz Mesmer. The doctor used conventional methods and began to explore magnets as the reason for relief.

The notion that internal fluids within the body could be controlled through magnets was "not outside the domain" of medical science that was well-known at the end of the 18th century. The most popular belief was that internal fluids could become externally "regulated" and hindered to benefit or harm. The theory had its beginnings in research papers by the scientist Sir Isaac Newton relating to gravitation.

Hypnosis is widely used in the present by medical scientists as a cure-all to a variety of phobias and problems. The habits of smoking, binge eating as well as mental disorders such as depression and sleep deprivation were solved after a couple of sessions.

It is often compared to meditation by some people who are not religious and also by people in general. The similarities aren't the same, in the sense that meditation doesn't have a specific goal in mind , aside from maybe the idea of an "inner peacefulness". Both methods are an in a state that is altered but if meditation is not a concentration, hypnosis allows for the possibility of "suggestions".

The suggestions are able to be modified in order to make them more beneficial for those looking to increase their wealth, health and overall well-being.

Dr. Mesmer was a consultant to many patients with psychiatric disorders, and managed to get some remarkable results. The term "mesmerism" remains connected to his name.

In in the late 19th century, it was clear that hypnotism began to lose its magical effects, and was the subject of research.

While the research of it could lead to the suicide of some doctors. It wasn't until beginning of the 20th century that the use of hypnotic suggestions at the start of surgery was considered as a legitimate method of operation.

The growing field of Psychiatry has proposed that the mind is overloaded with unfounded thoughts and thoughts. They can be managed through careful and thoughtful exercises.

The main goal in the exercises is to attain a "receptive awareness" or more sensitive "state in consciousness" which is distinct from the normal state. The state of hypnosis is described as watching an captivating film or it is experienced in Yoga or focusing on one's breathing.

The implication is that the person who is attracted to has been removed from their normal environment. In this state that thoughts are recited in monotonous tones. The conscious and the brain retain these signals, to respond to them and revisit painful memories or perhaps defending these last events, so the individual or patient can continue their journey.

Hypnotherapy finally was accepted in the AMA (American Medical Association) in 1958. certified practitioners were able to recommend the procedure to treat a variety of social problems, including controlling weight, alcohol abuse as well as anger management and other psychological problems.

Accredited by an established organization, hypnosis to benefit the general good has been used since the U.S. as well as Europe as well as some parts of the world that are developing. However, there are certain religious beliefs that ban its use, including those of the Christian Science, The Mormon Church as well as Jehovah's Witnesses. It is generally accepted by other religionsas it is advantageous to all races, colors and religions.

for good or bad

It is true that hypnotherapy is not without its negative side as well. It is not recommended for those suffering from psychosis severe or someone who is suffering from severe anti-social personality disorder because any suggestion that comes into their thoughts can put an individual into an emotional state. There are guidelines and rules that therapists must adhere to that do not infringe on the moral code of an individual during the process of hypnosis.

## Chapter 5: What Does It Mean?

To "Be Hypnotized?"

Apart from being an altered state of mind, hypnosis also a method. This is the natural and natural process that is designed to get you into a state of concentrated awareness where your mind becomes more open to positive suggestions understanding, insight, and awareness. In this state of focus that you can access your capacity to swiftly integrate new skills strategies, strengths, and insights, and also to let go of negative and ineffective thoughts, emotions and routines.

With your consent, authorization and as per your desire, a trained practitioner of hypnosis can assist you regain you back control in the areas where you feel out of control.

Regaining control over those unproductive, undesirable and unneeded thoughts, feelings and habits that hinder you from creating the life you've always wanted.

The only thing you need to meet for being hypnotized are consent and a desire. When you're engaged in self-hypnosis, or working with a professional, granting yourself permission to engage in the process, along with the intention of experiencing that is consistent with your objectives throughout and following the session is all you require to do to become hypnotized and the only thing you have to do to be able to enjoy the process completely.

It's like the subconscious choice we make when we decide to watch the latest movie. No matter whether we're watching it in a cinema or at the comfort at home, prior to starting the film, we've taken the decision to believe in our own eyes.

As if a small portion of us had not already decided to suspend our disbelief, to in a subliminal way realize that we've accepted our consent and have a want to "go through the motions" and experience all the emotions and experiences the film might bring us, we won't be able to overlook the fact that we're watching actors playing parts in a script written by someone else, and used speaking to cameras on a set that has been made up for a film that is set.

With that permission or desire we can become a part of the film and let ourselves feel all the feelings that actors and directors, producers, musicians, and cinematographers have directed us to.

We love the process and its results as well as the similar thing can happen when you are attempting to be controlled. An unforgettable experience that can have positive outcomes that can change your life!

What do you feel it feels like?

To be to be hypnotized?

Since hypnosis is a method that is unique to every person there's no one feeling that everyone experiences. There are a variety of common emotions which are experienced by all those who undergo hypnosis.

The majority of people report feeling relaxed and calm. It's possible to feel like you're sitting in your chair of choice after a long day. Many people find themselves in a relaxed flow while in hypnosis as if you're relaxing in a hammock during your well-deserved beach holiday.

Some people experience a sensation of relaxation, which has them feeling a heavy weight throughout their body as if they could not raise their arms, legs or even the eyelids even when they wanted to.

Others report experiencing the relaxation is a blissful sensation of light and floating like they're floating in the air in the chair they're in.

It's also not uncommon to feel nothing distinctive or unique during the course of time, instead, you'll feel like you're in a comfortable chair, listening to someone speak.

The varying experiences happen due to the fact that hypnosis isn't just about your body or the sensations you're experiencing, but an experience of mind, or the information you're processing in the subconscious.

When you go through hypnosis, you might experience different sensations at different intervals, and even during one session. It could be that you feel a sensation of relaxation in your legs, arms or even your body like you're sinking into the comfy position you're currently in. There may be a slight floating sensation as if you're floating over that place. It might feel like you're lying or sitting there in awe of every word spoken.

You may also find your thoughts drifting off and wandering away from spoken words to another place or thoughts.

All is normal and okay. What you feel is acceptable, as there's no specific feeling that is hypnotized.

In actual fact, during the hypnosis session, if you find yourself in the mood to move or scratch, swallow or change your position, you are at liberty to do that. It will allow you relax more.

Sometimes, you'll know precisely what's happening in the surrounding area and, always, of course, never giving the capacity to consider, think about, react and react in whatever way you think is appropriate.

Most people are convinced that they're not in a hypnosis , or that they're not doing anything wrong, since they're not thinking, still paying attention that they are still conscious. It is possible that you are your mind wandering over what you'll need to accomplish later... thinking about whether the noise is your stomach moving or people who hypnotize you... when your left hand is relaxed... and another thought that wander between your head. It's normal. It's your conscious mind doing what your conscious mind does - being aware and being conscious.

It is interesting to note that even though deep trance can feel amazing however, only a small amount of trance is needed to allow the work completed. We usually prefer the emotions physical and mental experienced by those in deep state of trance. It allows us to truly "check out" and enjoy a mental vacation. However, it's not required for changes. It's usually something that happens through the practice of it, but it's not an absolute requirement.

## Chapter 6: Are You Connected?

Establishing relationships and building relationships with others has been become an integral aspect of every day life. This is the one social skill that is essential at all times in every other aspect of our lives. We all are social creatures , and we require an individual who can understand us and be like us. This book because you wish that everyone would like you and want to establish a connection with them. Once you've started the process of understanding the human interaction and deciphering the secrets of how to influence people, I will ask two questions that I ask at the start of my workshops:

Q

How often did you feel an instant feeling of connection to the person whom you'd first met? When you first met that person, you'd feel like you've been with them for years. Have you ever met someone like this on your own?

Q

Have you lived or working with someone for years , and yet you aren't sure if you have any connection with that person?

Like my fellow participants in my trainings, I am sure that you've encountered those people in your daily lives. If I ask my students for why they felt attached to a particular person or why they felt they were not familiar with the person for them. I receive responses like:

I was able to connect to them since...

We also felt that way about certain aspects

He was truly kind and caring

They were very optimistic.

I was unable to connect due to...

I wasn't at ease with them.

I couldn't follow what they were saying.

Our wavelength didn't match

These are just a few of the numerous reasons you might or may not be able to connect in a particular manner with someone. Are you aware of the primary reason for why you think this way? The answer is quite simple. It is based on the relationship you develop with them. If you're not in connection with the person it is difficult to feel as if you're connected to them. it becomes difficult to develop the same chemistry. If you have a good relationship with someone, you instantly notice the chemistry that is present in your relationship.

In order to understand how to establish an effective relationship with the person you are talking to and create an emotional bond it is important to know the kind of people you meet. You will learn this in depth in the coming chapters. Prepare to write down notes and start working on the lessons.

People of different types

In the last chapter, I explained to you the reasons why you may feel a strong connection to someone you've just met , and also why you not feel as connected to a person who you've been in contact for a long time. The solution to this question was straightforward; it is based on the relationships you've built with them.

To make learning more engaging, I've made the decision to give an overview of how numerous types of people meet every day life. Once you have this information and are able to learn more about these characters.

If we talk about human beings in relation to their perception, there are three major types of people that you'll meet:

Visual person 2. Auditory person 3. Kinesthetic person

The three kinds of people each have their own unique way of communicating and comprehending things.

## Visual Person

A person who is visually dominant is the person who is more able to comprehend when they are presented to them through diagrams, graphs and pictures. The visual dominant person relies on their vision and imagination to convey their thoughts to the world. They depend on what they observe and how things appear to them. When they are thinking of something they instantly create images in their minds.

## Auditory Person

A person who is audiologist prefers paying attention to the content being taught to them. This can happen through presentations, voice recordings as well as group discussions. They view the world as it is presented to them or in accordance with the information they receive about it.

Kinesthetic Person

A person who is kinesthetic is the kind of person who likes to feel things both physically and emotionally. They are more inclined to experience things with hands and are more responsive to things with a touch or feel to them. When they imagine or think about things in their heads immediately, they associate the thought with feelings.

These are the three kinds of people we interact with. Understanding their traits can help you know how to handle them, and the way you must interact with them to maintain the bond between two of them.

Understanding the type of person is a crucial factor in all types of relationships, both professional and personal and helps you establish a connection and communicate with another person in a way that is generally recognized by the other person. There is a second series of questions I typically use in my seminars to highlight the importance of the type of person you're trying to establish a relationship with. My first question is...

A. What percentage of your readers been married?

If anyone has held their hands up, I request them to move to the side and form the group, and then I ask me a second question.

A. How how long are you married?

Some say one year, others say 5 years , and some give me 10 years and the list goes on. There is usually a mixed number of people in my classes and it makes it easy for me to demonstrate and communicate my message. The next question I have will be the one that makes the difference.

Question. Do you feel in love again with the one you're married to?

Then everyone in the group takes a moment to break and then responds with either a 'Yes' or'. I then take their permission and inquire as to what the reason for their response being one of 'yes' or'.

The people who gave me a positive response were very clear about the fact that they are still enjoying being together, and have discovered numerous similarities to their respective lives over the course of time, and so on.

After I had been asking the other participants, who had provided me with the opposite answer, the reason they don't feel romantically attached to their partners anymore they responded with questions such as:

There isn't a spark that remains between us

They don't act like they used to prior to marriage.

After my marriage, I realized that my spouse wasn't the right match for me.

My partner does not respond to me in the same way that she or he did at the beginning of our relationship.

The reasons I've given are just a some of the many reasons I learn about from the participants. What is the reason this occurs? The answer to this question was in the first chapter. section. Each person is one of three types, and when two types of people are paired up, they may aren't able to understanding one another in the end.

When you are in the initial phases of any relationship, no matter what type of the people you are and what kind of person you're dealing with typically, you often employ all three aspects to keep loved one you share with you amazed. The sensory channel and the visible channel, and finally the Kinesthetic channel. I will continue to discuss weddings in love for your ease of understanding.

If you are in love, the beginning of a relationship can be beautiful. You attempt to show your love for your spouse by telling them you appreciate them, giving them things they love and making gestures such as touching hands or hugging your loved one in your arms. Are you aware that you've unknowingly utilized the your visual channel (gift) or audio channel (saying I love you) and the kinesthetic channel (holding hands) and, consequently, whatever your partner is, they'll be amazed by you.

As the time passes by with your spouse You tend to use the primary channel for communicating your feelings of love and affection to your spouse. This leads to two situations.

You and your companion are of the same kind.

Your partner and you are two different kinds

It is not an issue if both participants are auditory, visual or Kinesthetic. The issue arises when the two partners are different. There are the following kinds of partnerships for the scenario 2:

Auditory - Visual

Visual - Kinesthetic

Auditory - Kinesthetic

Let's take the first couple as an illustration. The partner who is visual will do whatever they can in visual form to show their love however the person who hears is not as impressed by their efforts because their primary method of communication is aural. They like hearing the words that express their love for them, and that someone else likes them and would like to be in their company and the list goes on.

In this situation, couples begin to believe that they aren't the same anymore or the spark is gone, etc. The only way to resolve this is to figure out what kind of relationship you have with your partner and express your feelings in a manner that they can comprehend and easily perceive. This can strengthen your relationship and you'll be able to develop a stronger relationship and get to know one another. They will talk to you in the manner they comprehend the best and they'll are listening to everything you say.

The goal of this chapter was to help the reader understand why sometimes you struggle to make the other person comprehend the message you've given them. Knowing the type of person you're speaking to can help you determine the best way to communicate. they most comprehend and how they will respond.

This isn't just applicable to marriages and relationships It is also relevant in other types of relationships that which you are in with other people i.e. your are friends with your acquaintances, your family members and other such. It is also a crucial role in helping you identify the type of relationship you are sharing with the other person and how you should engage with them.

The main concern that comes to mind is: 'How can I tell which one is the other one The next chapters will help you understand more about it.

## Chapter 7: What is Hypnosis?

It's a question scientists in the main stream don't appear to be able to reach a consensus on, but there is one thing that is clear. It's not sleep, in fact, contrary to what they say. Sleep is mostly an unconscious state, whereas when you're hypnotized, you're truly in a level of awareness. It's possible to appear asleep, however you're actually not. Actually, the question is much easier to answer if we can dispel certain myths first. Here are some myths.

Only the weak-minded or weak willed individuals can be hypnotized. False, because to be hypnotized you must be focused and follow the instruction of your expert. Two features that aren't typically seen in people who are weak-willed or weak-minded.

It's simply relaxation. The majority of people who are in hypnosis will be quite relaxed, and possibly more relaxed than what they remember feeling prior to the experience. But it's not the case that hypnosis can be described as relaxing. It is possible to be in hypnosis but not feel at all relaxed. In some cases, during hypnotherapy, the client might react, a term that is used to describe a person who is experiencing distress, perhaps recalling a traumatizing incident. How can one be relaxed when recalling a traumatizing incident? If you're not at ease, remember that you can benefit from hypnosis but without feeling at ease.

The hypnotist is in way too much power over me. The real control lies with the individual who is being at the receiving end of the hypnosis. Hypnosis is dependent on the person being hypnotized to trust the person being hypnotised, when you are convinced that the hypnotist is trying to make you perform something that you don't want to do, you will not let yourself be hypnotized. If you are feeling under hypnosis, that the hypnotist has crossed boundaries that you would prefer not, you'll instantly be released from hypnosis and your faith with the individual has been shattered. In addition, your critical faculty, and I'll talk about the critical faculty in the future and will not permit you to follow instructions that are against your moral or ethical code of conduct.

It is difficult to remember what happened. A small percentage of people , this may be true but it's very difficult to find and therefore affects just one or two people. Most people will recall certain things, but only a few people recalling all of the things. There's no way of knowing which category you fall into, but , as I've mentioned, the majority of people can remember certain.

It's not exactly natural. People are often surprised how natural it seems. It is a common occurrence for us to enter naturally occurring trances each day. It's likely that you've been in one these trances and you realize that you're at the next junction on the motorway. However, you don't recall your last twenty miles that seem to have flown by in a flash. You're in a trance when you're watching something on television and nothing else attracts your attention. You're not at risk because your subconscious will be in charge of its primary job to take care of you and protect you.

It's just all junk from the new age. What is your definition of "new age" since if that it's been around for at least a few millennia, then it's a new age. It was utilized by ancient Egyptians and also in the Far East for health and medical reasons for a long time long. It's been utilized within The Far East, it just was not widely used with the West until the time of Franz Anton Mesmer's time at the end of the 1800s. Mesmer is believed to have observed an Catholic priest known as Father Johann Gassner, who used methods of hypnosis for exorcisms with an Crucifix. Mesmer didn't believe in evil spirits were involved, however, he believed that the crucifix was magnetized. Based on this, he proceeded to create his theory of animal magnetism. In 1884, Abbe Faria resisted Mesmer's theory of animal magnetism. He presented Mesmer's patients were in fact treatment was not due to the magnets they used, but through the suggestions offered. Because of Mesmer's acclaim, Faria was ignored. He was absolutely right Magnetism was not the only factor in common with Mesmer's fame. Dr. James Esdaile performed over 400 operations while in India with the hypnosis method. His account in an medical journal was disregarded out of hand because it was believed "whereas this procedure might be suitable for an Indian but we wouldn't consider it suitable for an European or a Britisher". The bigoted view was disproved by Dr. John Elliotson performed successful operations in front of 200 doctors. In the short background, you can see that evidence that this isn't true and it is.

After dispelling some myths, and we're now able to discuss what exactly hypnosis is. There's multiple definitions used by hypnotists based on their personal preferences, not differing understandings of what hypnosis means therefore I'll present two options and let you decide by yourself which you would prefer. The first is that "it is a state that is elevated of suggestion". This definition is interpreted as being true due to the factors that make it efficient. Tips given during the state of hypnosis are more likely to affect than suggestions given while not in the state of hypnosis. The other definition would be "the removal from this Critical Faculty". I've already have mentioned that the Critical Faculty before and to be able to comprehend this definition, it is necessary to know what it means. What is the Critical Faculty, I'll just refer to it as the CF from this point on The CF is similar to a bouncer at nightclubs to the subconscious. The primary job that the unconscious has is to ensure that you are alive and secure, so it has its own view of the world. It isn't interested in being confused or to have its views be questioned. This could lead to fatal consequences. The views you have held keep you awake to date, so they're the most secure viewpoint. This is the place where the CF comes in. The CF will only take into the subconscious thoughts that conform to "known reality". Like the bouncer who was told not to let people in who are not wearing shoes. If a customer attempts to gain entry by wearing running shoesbut they do not conform to the appropriate shoes that are allowed into. The bouncer blocks admission. If you think that all spiders are dangerous, and you're shown a photograph of a spider, and are told "this one is secure" then the CF will immediately deny this notion and the false belief persists. If you're in a hypnotic state. In a hypnotic state, the CF is ignored and the thought goes straight to the subconscious. The subconscious is bypassing the CF that old, incorrect beliefs that cause the behavior that we'd like to change are put in the correct or more recent context. Another definition is "a hyper-focus and focus". In order to when you enter a hypnotic state, it is necessary to focus and concentrate on your instructions. This one is fairly easy to understand.

Hypnotherapists will explain that it is self-hypnosis. It is due to the focus required by the person who is hypnotizing. The hypnotherapist cannot force you to focus or force you to think of what they have to say during the hypnotic introduction. It is your choice to follow the instructions, as a result, you will be able to claim that you're hypnotizing yourself. The client is completely in control over the process and is able to stop it at any time they wish to. Keep in mind that no hypnotist could actually force you to do something you do not want to do or do anything that violates your own moral code.

I've been asked if the degree of hypnosis be quantified. It can be measured in a certain degree. It's not the intensity of hypnosis being assessed, but rather the impact it has on the brainwaves. The hypnotherapist may not possess the necessary equipment to measure the brainwaves of your patients and therefore is relying upon visual cues. Using Electroencephalography EEG it is possible to see brainwave activity. Brainwaves that are measured between 15 and 40 Hz (beta waves) indicate a mind that is active perhaps engaged in conversation, but conscious. Since brain waves decrease I frequency to 9 or 14 Hz (Alpha waves) the mind isn't as active, and Alpha waves are linked to an energised or relaxed state of mind. The brainwaves are then brought down to 4-8 cycles per second (Theta waves) This is the frequency range the brainwaves go through when we sleep or in a trance state of mind. Memory that is suppressed can be accessed during that frequency band. It can also be the range of frequency that brainwaves take place when we enter one of our everyday naturally occurring hypnotic Trances. If a brainwave frequency between one to four Hz (Delta waves) is detected, then you've been in the most lucid state of relaxation that is possible, with an average of 2-3 Hz recorded in sleep that is obviously isn't an hypnotic state.

Whatever definition you like is completely yours to decide, but the most important thing to remember is that hypnosis is able to bring about swift and powerful modifications in a completely safe and natural manner. Hypnotherapy and hypnosis isn't an all-purpose solution or magic wand that can cure-all. It can assist you in bringing changes, but you need to desire that change. There's no reason to go to a hypnotherapist and telling them to that you must quit smoking since your partner has told you to since your partner is trying to convince you to quit smoking. In this case, it will not perform and any professional hypnotherapist isn't going to invest your money and put it in false hope that you will make to change your lifestyle. According to the old joke How many hypnotherapists do need to replace the bulb in a lightbulb? Only one , and the light bulb must be a desire to be changed.

The First Consultation

If you decide to book an hypnotherapist, prior to them begin working on your issues, they will require certain details. This information is collected during the initial meeting. Although no therapeutic hypnosis will take place during this consultation, it is a crucial session for both hypnotherapists and clients alike. Hypnotherapists, like me, want to customize their clients' sessions with hypnotherapy. Personalising the hypnotherapy session makes them more effective and can bring lasting change much easy to attain in comparison to the general one-size-fits-all sessions. To the casual observer, this data gathered might seem completely irrelevant to the issue that the client is trying to resolve. There will be questions about names of children and their ages along with the names of your partners and their ages as well as jobs (yours and those of your companions) as well as information on relatives and friends. It is possible that you feel that these topics are not relevant but it allows us to tailor your sessions to ensure greater satisfaction.

During this time , your use in a language is scrutinized. Your language use can be a significant indicator to your method of treatment. This information is used to create the words of your sessions with therapists to increase their effectiveness.

Another crucial aspect of the initial consultation is that it's your opportunity to ask questions regarding the hypnotherapy and hypnosis. However, this doesn't mean you can't ask questions later on however it's an ideal moment to inquire. It's the ideal moment to seek answers to your questions. It's because you're becoming acquainted with the hypnotherapist before deciding if you are able to trust them. Be aware that if you aren't confident in the hypnotherapist or are skeptical about hypnosis it is unlikely that hypnosis will be conducted. Therefore, ask questions regarding all aspects of hypnosis. It's also a good moment to inquire regarding their level of training.

You might be asked to sign a formal contract agreeing to hypnosis. I personally will always talk about the number of sessions needed and the time we examine your improvement. Before the beginning of each session I talk with you about how much improvement has occurred in the past session. This is the stage that we might decide to extend the duration of sessions or to reduce the amount of sessions as necessary. Some might argue that it's just a means to increase the number of sessions and making more money from the clientele, but the reality is that this kind of behavior is harmful to any practice of hypnotherapy. People who have been harmed by this type of conduct aren't likely to refer their friends and family members and in fact, they may stop them from seeing the hypnotherapist, and therefore it is sensible for any hypnotherapist to bring a client in for the smallest amount of sessions needed for the transformation the client desires. It's equally likely that the amount of sessions will decrease rather than increased. Therefore, you pay less for sessions and the hypnotherapist will maintain a an excellent reputation in the profession and both of them benefit. Any increase or decrease in session length should be negotiated by both the hypnotherapist as well as the client.

If you've never been previously hypnotised and you have the time certain hypnotherapists can with your permission conduct an induction that is hypnotic and hypnotize you. It serves three reasons. It provides the client with an experience of the trance hypnotic experience like and provides an idea of what to expect while in a state of trance. This is also a chance to provide the new customer, with consent an after hypnotic suggestion to allow the hypnotherapist use to initiate the session quickly on the very first session of therapy. Another benefit is that the client is able to go to their personal space without wasting time during therapy sessions. They may even receive instructions to, when it's suitable to take a break and relax in their home or place of refuge between the first consultation and the therapy session. This will enable the client to experience going to a state of relaxation. Keep in mind that we all learn better by practicing.

It is possible that you are wondering whether you'll be charged for the first consultation. This is contingent on the hypnotherapist who is in question. Some do not charge for the first consultation because there is no therapy taking place. Others do charge. The cost is usually less than a therapeutic session however it's one hour of their time used, which isn't able to be transferred on to other clients. There's always the possibility that you will not be able to schedule any therapeutic sessions, or that the hypnotherapist might feel that you're not suitable for therapy with hypnosis. In such cases, the hypnotherapist may have invested hours of their time but does not schedule a session with a client, and a lot of hypnotherapists believe that it's only fair to get some benefit from the initial consultation. We're all trying to earn an income, and offering our time in exchange for free time doesn't seem right.

Different Suggestions

There are three basic types of suggestion that are used in the field of hypnotherapy. The direct suggestion. This kind of suggestion is essentially an instruction. It's used to instruct you to take action. "Close the eyes" is a common induction technique. could be a direct request. There's also the indirect suggestion where people's subconscious who is being hypnotized determines when and how to perform the induction. A typical example of this during an induction could be similar to "When the eyes of your at ease close your eyes. Your eyes will be able to tell when it's time to close them, so let them close when they're prepared". This allows power to your subconscious, whereas direct suggestion is a way to control over the magician. There is no way to say that one of these kinds of suggestions is superior to one for every person. A majority of people be more responsive to one or one, it's a it's a matter of the hypnotherapist figuring out what is the best approach for you. We refer to this as you modality. You can choose between two modality however , and the hypnotherapist is able to determine the best way to structure your sessions, linguistically according to the type of modality you are using. Another type of suggestion is known as the post-hypnotic suggestion. These are suggestions that are designed to be executed in the same way as they sound after the hypnotherapy session has ended and you're no more in a state of trance. This is possible to use it to fix the behavior or help achieve an outcome you want to achieve. A good example is such as "When you are bored, think about that instead of eating a snack, you can take an hour-long walk or read the book. A snack won't alleviate your boredness". This is a good example for a person who has a tendency to eat out of boredom and needs motivation to exercise, and has pointed out a different way of doing things that is not snacking, such like reading. The subconscious is presented with the option of activities that were highlighted in previous sessions to be activities that are more enjoyable than having a snack.

## Chapter 8: Regression Methods

In an "direct suggestion" method of therapy, the therapist is able to perform"regres(or regressive) procedure.

The following are the main points:

"Feel the emptyness in your stomach. Feel that empty feeling increasing in strength.

Feel the sensation grow so intense that you feel it stronger than before. (Implosive Technique). When you feel this empty feeling growing stronger and more powerful, let your

self to return in time. .... Now, go back to the very first moment in your life you've ever experienced this

The feeling of being empty. Now think back to the first time you felt this ..."

Repeat this procedure until your subject is able to recall the incident in their life that triggered the incident.

resulted in a personal experience of disapproval, absence of love or attention, or that which what it was that made it synonymous with emptyness. Keep going until you find out the time

The need to satisfy an emotional desire was satisfied by food consumed on behalf of the subject. At an era

Your subject has substituted food to fill up the void in the hope of finding satisfaction. You

It is often found that the root reason for obesity is usually an absence of attention, love or affection for an

young age.

Your client could have parents who were alcoholics, and they might have hit, yelled at, or other

The perpetrators of great and a lot of. Your only hope is that your subject would feel secure or safe is to ensure that they are secure.

was to fill your stomach up with foods, but preferably sweets or candy because "Granny

always had candy for me often. Granny always was the sole person who loved me."

If your loved one realizes that she has turned to food in exchange for love, she is able to

Then, you can separate them and see that attention, love, and affection are supplied by the one you love

Ones that are not food, but ones that are not food. Your patter could sound like this: "You now know that friends, loved ones family, relatives and others provide you with

Attention, love and affection. Now you realize that you're not in that circumstance and

You aren't living to the days of old and you do not have to substitute foods for anything

emotional turmoil you felt the emotional turmoil you experienced at the emotional turmoil you experienced at that. It will be apparent that you are now loved by someone you once loved.

loved ones, family and friends members who completely meet your emotional needs and

Foods satisfy only your body's needs for health and nutrition. The body will no longer require any

interest in sweets, fattening items, etc....etc....."

What you've done is allow your subject to eliminate the unconscious

the idea that food can have something to do with satisfying the needs of our emotions. If this is the case, then

done, your work accomplished will be much more easy. By regressing, accomplished your work will be much easier.

This has allowed your client to discover the true reason of the eating disorder initially

and to implement mental correction actions that result in permanent clarity

of the issue.

In some instances, your subject won't be facing an issue with substitution, but will be making use of

weight loss to avoid potential prospective suitors. She argues that so long as she's overweight , she will

Not attractive, therefore isn't a risk for sexual interaction. It is evident that this is a type of

The client can take weight off initially using directly suggested suggestion, and afterwards, it will be put back on

with a dramatic change when she is close to her level of insecurity regarding her sexuality. When she's close to her point of insecurity,

If the fundamental issue isn't dealt by you, you'll get short-term results.

You can also employ the implosive method if you notice that she is experiencing any of the following

sensation that is associated with the desire eating. But, you might have take a different approach

to support her back until she's slim and not having any difficulties in gaining the weight. Graduation

You can bring her to the point that she began putting on pounds:

"Now, Mary, you are twenty-two...you are two and declare that you are

You are beginning to begin to. Now you're in the exact moment that you begin to eating more. What's the matter?

What are you currently doing? What do you do, Mary, that makes you want to eat more?"

(Allow for her to find the reason, and then proceed in the separation process to allow the subject is able to distinguish her sexual desires from sublimated by food.)

The situation could be challenging since the cause could be due to of

poor relationship. She might be aware of the root of her issues, but is unwilling to seek out a solution

of the marriage and , consequently, of the marriage and refusing to let go of any weight, irrespective of

whatever efforts the therapist makes. If it is the case even if you're not an a

A licensed marriage counselor may suggest counseling for families and marriage

Your client must wait until she is able to meet her own requirements and wants to shed the excess weight in line with.

A second factor that you'll often encounter is that of the "role model" factor. A lot of

Little girls grow up with overweight mothers who do not make an effort to lose weight , and encourage

the child who is overweight is normal to be overweight as they grow older. Other aspects include

"manliness", "big man", "big and strong" and other incorrect images chosen

beginning in the early years of childhood, which promotes being in the early years that encourage being overweight.

The legendary comic Jackie Gleason was treated by Dr. William J. Bryan, Jr. in

Los Angeles, California for obesity. Doctor. Bryan was successful in aiding Mr. Gleason shed weight, but in losing weight, Jackie did not become "funny". Jackie believed that he needed to

overweight to appear "funny". Jackie maintained his weight while he was a TV comic. He was able

He did shed weight, but he was unable to lose weight each time this he felt anxious about his job and put
the weight back onto.

## Chapter 9: The Model

Being called hypo-therapist is similar to being called para-trooper! A para-trooper is an individual soldier who travels to where the need is by with a parachute. The parachute. Therefore, the word para in para-trooper is a reference to the system of delivery utilized. It is the same that hypnotherapy is merely a method of delivery for therapy. What I am referring to is that for any therapist, the most crucial thing will always be employing the most effective treatment available to them. The delivery method is enjoyable and can provide benefits to using pills that go beyond what is stated in the label of the pills. However, I am not going to reveal about the advantages of hypnosis are. That will be revealed through knowledge.

Hypnosis is among the most effective methods available to create positive change in people. to help you achieve this, I'll attempt to give you an easy and effective method. The method we'll use here is a single method of hypnosis, but it is however it is not the only method. This is the method I employ to use the hypnosis method and covers all the information you require to help hypnosis function.

The model we'll be working on looks like the following 1. Pre-talk.

Step 2: Test for suggestibility.

Step 3 Induction.

Step 4: Intensify-er.

Step 5 First suggestions.

Step 6: Make suggestions.

Step 7 7. Closure.

Step 8: Termening the session.

Each step is an entire chapter to itself and any doubts or frequently-asked questions I receive are answered.

The aim of the book is to give an essential set of tools, within a framework which allows you to utilize hypnosis as a tool for marketing, therapy, and entertainment. In order to do this, we will teach one test of suggestibility, one induction, and a deeperener. This will allow you to master one test, induction and deepener effectively instead of several poorly, and further every test sequence, including induction, and deepener can be incorporated into the framework we provide.

There are numerous inductions available on YouTube that which you can download free of charge. The same is true for the tests for suggestibility. You can learn and test each one at a time and after a few weeks they will run through your head.

This section of Q&A is in the last section because you'll get more information from it once you understand how it is done. This isn't a collection of scripts, but with this book you can construct your own scripts that are based on the client's questions and comprehension.

# Chapter 10: Understanding Hypnosis

Hypnosis is used by millions of people over many thousands of years. It has been proven to decrease stress, increase sleeping patterns, enhance your body and relieve pain, or even get rid of bad habits such as smoking and eating too much.

Many people view it as something unusual it is actually a normal experience that everybody has experienced. One instance of a natural state of hypnosis is what's commonly referred to as "highway hypnosis" or being at a state of hypnosis by the road while you drive. Once you have arrived at the destination, you don't recall driving or even having seen the normal landmarks. You were in a state, and you left your motoring to the "automatic driver."

The same hypnotic state can be experienced when you're too involved in a novel, movie or television show or other task that you shut out all other distractions. It's so intense with what you're doing that if someone walks into the room and wants to speak to you, it's impossible to hear or see the person. This is also a typical state of hypnosis. When you focus that intensely it is easy to slip into this natural hypnotic condition.

The term "hypnos" is an Greek word that literally translates to "to to sleep." However, hypnosis is distinct from sleeping. It's not even close to sleep since your brain is constantly alert.

A state of hypnosis can be described by intense suggestibility, relaxation, and an increased imagination. It is often compared with dreaming or the sensation that you are "losing your self" in the pages of a novel or film. It is a state of consciousness however, you are unable to focus on the majority of the world surrounding you.

The hypnotic experience by itself is only beneficial in promoting relaxation it is essential to ensure that the mind remains open and responsive to suggestions to heal and change your emotional state.

Myths about Hypnosis

The word "hypnosis" is associated with images of stage hypnotists who encourages their audience to quack like ducks, cluck as chickens or play the guitar like Elvis or make fun of themselves in one way or some other manner. You've probably watched the TV or film hypnotist that seems to be able of curing any illness and solve any issue, all using the ability of their own strong mind.

There are those who believe that hypnotism can be an evil art form that could be used to take control of someone else's mind as a form of brainwashing employed for all kinds of criminality. There are also those who aren't convinced of hypnosis in any way in any way.

With all the theories and contradictory information It's no wonder that people are confused what exactly hypnosis is?

The Truth about Hypnosis

Hypnotism is a type of persuasion. In reality, hypnotism is sometimes described in the context of "the technique of persuasion." According to me it's a true description. When hypnotized the person being in a state of hypnosis is persuaded something is real. The truth could be that they're not interested in an additional cigarette, or that they're an animal.

Usually, when someone tries convincing you to believe that something's real then you'll reject the notion unless presented with solid proof. This is why, regardless of how convincing they appear they are, no one can convince you that you're an innocent chicken.

You're not likely convince someone you're chickens unless they actually would like to be a chicken or are already persuasive. The use of hypnosis may be utilized to "nudge" the mind of a person in the event that they're willing with the concept.

How Hypnosis works

How do you convince an individual to believe something that they might not believe? Although there are different methods of doing it The main goal is to put yourself "under the radar" through direct communication with the person's subconscious mind.

One of the easiest methods is to make the person to feel relaxed and at ease. This lets them drop their guards and fall into an "suggestible situation." This state is where, with the correct words the person who hypnotizes "leads" them to the desired outcome. With careful wording the hypnotist lays out subtle concepts in a manner that allows the individual to recognize (rather than to reject) the result. When they come back from a hypnotic state they tend to accept the concepts to become their own.

# Chapter 11: Hypnosis Mp3s - A Technology Advantage

Therapy for Hypnotherapy: Past, Present, and Future

The background of hypnotherapy is fascinating, but it is well outside the limits of this article. Here are some interesting facts

Utilizing hypnosis for the treatment of psychological problems and in managing pain during childbirth and during surgery was recognized by the British Medical Association as long in 1955. The BMA at the time recommended that all physicians and medical students must receive a basic education in the art of hypnosis.

In 1956 in 1956, it was in the year 1956 that the Roman Catholic Church - which up until that point had explicitly banned the practice of using hypnosis approved its use for the diagnosis and treatment of certified health care experts.

In 1958 in 1958, the American Medical Association approved the therapeutic uses of hypnosis, and encouraged more research.

In 1960 in 1960, in 1960, the American Psychological Association endorsed hypnosis as a psychology-related field.

It is apparent that, although stage hypnotists have been on the news but hypnotherapists are in the shadows and quietly working within private practices for a long time.

As I've seen in the books I've read, first pre-recorded hypnosis session was created and sold in the year 1976 in the year 1976 by American Hypnotherapist Dick Sutphen. These were audio cassette tapes.

Cassette tapes were eventually replaced in the 1990s with compact disks (CDs). Numerous hypnotherapists continue to offer recorded hypnosis sessions pre-recorded on CDs for those who want that alternative.

There's an advancement in technology that makes it simpler than ever before for hypnotherapists provide their expertise to the general public (and consequently help more people outside of their offices) This technology is known as MP3.

MP3s can compress enormous quantities of data to an even smaller size which means it's now possible to transfer large and more sophisticated pre-recorded, sessions of hypnosis from one computer to another over the internet. You're probably used to using MP3s to listen tracks and songs.

MP3s are quick to download, easy to use, and compatible with a range of devices , including Apple iTunes, Windows Media Player, RealPlayer, the iPod, Microsoft Zune and mobile phones.

The Main Advantages Hypnosis MP3s

There is no doubt that, in certain situations, particularly deeply rooted problems traditional face-to-face hypnotherapy is the best choice. The ability of a practitioner to read and respond immediately to non-verbal or spoken responses from clients throughout the hypnotic process is crucial in certain situations, but this isn't something that is possible to replicate in a recorded hypnosis session.

In the majority of cases the majority of cases, we don't necessarily require the attention of an experienced practitioner. We just need their talents and knowledge to assist us achieve something for ourselves which is why an appropriate and effective Hypnosis MP3 is the best solution.

The greatest benefit of using hypnosis MP3s is that they do not require me to acquire new techniques. They are simple and easy to using, and also to get the greatest rewards with the least effort, nothing is better than their performance. They are the closest thing you can get to having someone else take on all the tasks.

Maybe for many people, the initial attraction of a pre-recorded digital sessions of hypnosis would be one of the biggest benefits - its cost.

My own study of the charges imposed by more than 70 different hypnotherapists found that the median cost for one face-to-face session in person was $156.

So far that hypnotherapists generally are of the opinion that most issues require between three to eight sessions to be resolved. Based on these numbers that a typical series of live session with a professional hypnotherapist may cost anything from $400 to over $1200.

But, when an hypnotherapist designs a typical or complete session for all the typical issues he or she faces in private practice, and then offers sessions as recordings using the most affordable method that is available, what's the cost of a session today?

For one hypnosis MP3 I've spent as little as $8.95 and as high as $19.95.

It's not much of a commitment to finance, is it?

Here are some additional benefits of hypnosis. MP3s:

You control the experience. You're at your home and can press the play button whenever you want to.

There's no need to choose the top local hypnotherapist and you can select your hypnotherapist among the top in the world.

It's not necessary to schedule your schedule to meet with the local hypnotherapist, or travel to the office of your hypnotherapist and all the extra time required. Listen to the hypnosis MP3s at any time and wherever it will suit your needs.

You get instant access to your preferred expert's skills and talents when you're inspired to make favorable changes for yourself. You can buy the hypnosis MP3 immediately online, download it right away and enjoy all the advantages of listening in just a few minutes.

You have unlimited access to the hypnotherapist's expertise and skills. You can listen to audio hypnosis recordings as often as you want or need to and repeat sessions do not add up to the price as the subsequent sessions of face-to face therapy do. In reality it's a cost for the initial session, and each session following which is completely absolutely free.

There are some therapeutic "side outcomes' of listening to the hypnosis MP3s. Particularly, you are able to experience relaxation naturally. A lot of people don't know how to relax themselves naturally, or how to truly relax. Relaxation can also help reduce stress, which according to the source you choose is responsible for between 75% to 95% of all physical ailments.

Hypnosis MP3s are secure and provide security. Listening to them on headphones or earphones. Nobody is aware of what you're listening to other than you. This is a great option for those who are just beginning to learn about Hypnosis, especially if they have in your family and people who aren't willing to support your enthusiasm. Hypnosis MP3s are great for those who don't wish to talk about their problems with a real-life professional or anyone else.

Hypnosis MP3s cover an extensive variety of subjects and in the same way that the more traditional topics are expanding into increasingly specific sub-topics, and new topics are added constantly and expanded, there are more opportunities for us to become more precise with our use of hypnosis MP3s. They can help us find the right fit for us and what we are looking for each time.

The top quality hypnosis MP3s sound so excellent that when your eyes have closed you'll probably notice not much difference between listening to the hypnotherapist's voice in the convenience of your own home, and sitting in their consulting room.

The advancements in digital technology are creating it possible to include features in the hypnotic recordings that go that go beyond what could normally be present in live in-person hypnotherapy. A few producers of hypnosis MP3s are playing in the present to determine how beneficial this opportunity could be.

The Hypnosis Habit is a way to develop
Repetition is an essential component of all pre-recorded sessions with hypnosis. Through consistency and persistence, we can attain our goals and all it needs to be

done is the development of a habit of listening.

The majority of hypnosis MP3s are standalone single sessions that you can listen to daily when they're related to goals (until your goal has been met) or any other time you're able to.

Some products for hypnosis have several sessions. As an example, there may be an introduction session to get the listener acquainted with the effects of hypnosis (which typically only needs to listen to only once) and the main hypnosis session that focuses on the subject you are interested in and possibly an alternate version or additional session that is that is related to the same topic.

Some other hypnosis programs are more of a sequence of MP3s. Some of that are hypnosis sessions, and others are audios that contain pertinent information and tips that can be listened to while "awake". I typically refer to these as "programs". They usually cover major areas of change , such as smoking cessation or weight loss where psychological assistance may frequently be required.

For both the multiple-session hypnosis product as well as the hypnosis software, the hypnotherapist usually provides you with directions or suggestions on how and when to listen to each of the MP3s.

Also, there are what is commonly called "bundles". They are hypnosis sessions that are just one with related topics that are offered at a discounted cost. For instance, it could be an "Health and Fitness" package of say six hypnosis session with subjects like healthy cooking, slimming your body or whatever it may be. The cost is lower than if you purchased each session individually.

The hypnotherapist will generally give directions or tips regarding how and when to listen to each of the MP3s.

According to my experience, there's no benefit in having the same hypnosis sessions at least once a day.

Making Results

The issue of how long it'll be to get a desired outcome using a hypnosis MP3 difficult to answer. In fact it is unlikely to have any one solution.

It is possible to get the desired result with just one session of hypnosis?

It is true, especially when what we desire is simply a change in the way we perceive. For instance, I utilize Hypnosis MP3s to help with problem solving, breaking out of the cycle of thinking as well as to reduce stress, and other similar reasons. And, in these instances I typically employ a particular MP3 only when required. Hypnosis is great for these kinds of scenarios.

If our goal is altering our behavior patterns but that isn't enough, it calls for a different kind of application.

I have seen numbers that are quoted to show the time it takes to alter the habit (or more precise, to change an existing habit to a brand new habit) and they are somewhat random. It could take 21 days or the equivalent of 28 days or 90 days, as an example. Maybe, if the level of change needed is higher the process will take longer than it does.

In my experience of creating new habits, there are generally many variables at the mix to make a precise prediction.

For instance What is the behavior I'm trying to change imprinted in my childhood or is it simply an "bad" habit that I taken on during my adulthood which I'd love to rid myself of?

Do I use an MP3 hypnosis as a stand-alone method or is it being used in conjunction with a different personal growth technique or other life-style changes?

Are you really driven to get the result you have stated you would like or are you just trying to please others?

It's crucial to differentiate between obtaining results and generating changes.

Change begins the moment you make the decision to change and it can happen even when we believe it's not, therefore you shouldn't be dissatisfied when, as often happens, a hypnosis treatment hasn't had any effect at all.

There have been times that I've listened to new hypnosis MP3 for myself and had to listen to at least two or three sessions before I was able to be aware of fresh thoughts on the topic of interest. That could be normal.

Proper responses to the suggestions of a hypnotherapist may be happening initially in a state of unconscious.

It is possible to see a change in a flash, and may take a couple of days to reach the outcome you want, or one week, or even a month, or even longer. It all depends on the goal is.

As you go, pay attention to the things you observe. Evidence that your mind is guiding you towards the desired result will come to light So be on the lookout for even the smallest of things you're not doing as.

Although hypnosis MP3s are as powerful as they could be, I believe that, besides those instances that do require an alteration in our perspective, "instant success" is not a realistic expectation of the technology. In order to develop new habits, and more sophisticated uses of hypnosis, repeated use of a recorded hypnosis program is likely to be required and we should expect that to be the case. However, certain situations will require more repetition than other issues in any case.

In most cases, and dependent on the type of music that you're playing, the period during which you can be sure to get the results you want is suggested by the hypnotherapist , and that's always something to keep an eye on and be assured by.

Visualization

Mental imagery is usually defined as the language spoken by our subconscious mind. The better we're in imagining during hypnosis the more potent our experience as well as the more profound impact it has on our thoughts and emotions, as well as our subsequent behavior.

Typically, when we carry on with the tasks of our lives and work, we're in a highly and focused on the outside and don't pay attention to our mental images in any way. This could be a problem in the beginning when we're not used to being in a state of hypnosis and realize the ability of our brain to see isn't well-developed.

Effective visualization I believe that effective visualization is it's an acquired skill and is something that people require to develop and develop. In my experience, improvement will occur naturally as a result of regular exercise.

There is also the so-called "imaginary" using the five physical senses. When we are thinking of things in general, or are requested to think of something specific, for instance in hypnosis that is not our normal sense of sight could dominate. For instance, smells and sounds, for instance, could in many instances be more vivid and evocative to something that's "imaginary" experience than what we be able to see.

If visualization seems to be an issue for you, believe that, with repetition and practice, your visualization will grow more powerful . And even when your mental images aren't evident, the sense of what you're required to consider will suffice.

Multiple Projects

Do not try to alter everything in your life all at once.

It's a big mistake. We've all been there. You could end up spending much of your time doing things which are no not more that superficial.

It's much better to remain focussed and patient. It is a good idea to keep a vision in your head of your ideal lifestyle. While you're at it you can make small improvement each day, and then a year in the future ... Who will know? Five years from today? You could be amazed. Take a stroll by taking baby steps and continuing forward motion.

It might be beneficial to prioritize the positive changes you wish to bring about within your own life, and then begin with what is the most important or urgent to you today.

My experience is that the amount of tasks which hypnosis could help you to accomplish is determined by the opportunities available to you in your everyday life to listening to the hypnosis MP3s.

Even under ideal conditions it is not advisable for you to go through more than three MP3s of hypnosis each day, as if you attempt to listen to more than that , you'll begin to lose your focus.

The hypnosis audios you listen to do not necessarily come from the same professional. As with me, you might find a specific hypnotherapist that best suits your needs generally. However, there will be times where he or she can't provide exactly what you're looking for, so you'll have to find a different professional who can provide it.

In the event that you listen to more than one MP3 per day it's not a good option listening to these in a row even if the topics are related. When you're dealing with more than three MP3s of hypnosis, they should be being listened to in three or two separate intervals of time. If you're only able to find enough time to dedicate one hour or so to your meditation MP3s , and you're using more than one of them, make sure you take an interval of at least five minutes following a session to let your thoughts calm before starting the next session.

# Chapter 12: How to Become a Hypnotist

What? Are you not already an hypnotist, but you desire to take to the to the stage? You're certainly a fit for a straight-jacket , if that is the situation.

Do you? If you are a novice to nothing about hypnosis, then you're likely to have less to learn than those who have been practicing the practice for a long time. You could stay clear of some of the negative naysaying that is prevalent in the world of therapy training in which stage hypnosis is not good, and hypnotism is apparently doing not do anyone any favors, and is said to cast negative image of hypnotherapy generally.

However in the event that you've had the hypnotherapy course or you're self-taught and are looking to add a new strings to the bow of your hypnosis the stage hypnosis technique will increase your confidence, provide you with some new methods and expand the client base of your business of therapy. Even if some trainers in hypnotherapy declare that stage hypnosis can be undesirable, does not mean it's not.

The art of hypnotising isn't really the focus in this publication. I will mention some excellent books and training courses in the final chapter as well as some further explanations of terms and concepts that are included in the show section of the book. However, I would strongly recommend that if you do not have any previous experience with hypnosis, to begin with online courses or read a few books and progress from there. It is not difficult to learn hypnosis and neither is getting skilled with the technique (especially with proper education) However, it's a skill that requires a lot of words to impart properly. I'd like to keep this book as short and accessible.

Like I've stated in the past, go to the websites and read the books, take the basics of training, and return when you're ready to move on to your next stage.

Pre-Show

The show does not begin until the music begins and you step onto the stage. It must start prior to your grand entry. Your audience should be aware that they're coming to an event that is stage-hypnosis. They should be aware that they're going to be entertained, will be entertained as they have the risk of being entertainment, and that they are safe while they're doing it. You must create this expectation, particularly prior to when you are branded by the title of THE Hypnotist. (Every stage performer is THE Hypnotist since if they're not they're not going to give the audience what they deserve).

The expectations can be created by a variety of methods - the stunning poster of youwith your fingers spread out and your arms placed at eye level , and pointed at a woman in her 20s who appears to be is beginning to slide back. It could seem like a cliché however it is effective and is understood by your target audience. Your website should include videos of your show and the website address should be included in every piece of marketing that you release. A press release sent to the local newspaper , talking in hyperbole about the previous show. A radio interview in which an assistant to the production (never the primary presenter) is required to speak in bizarre dialects live on air, or respond in a sloppy manner to any question, or engage in similar insanity that causes the presenter to laugh, that creates the possibility of entertainment in the minds of the viewers. It is essential that they know that they're going to see an hypnotist in case they don't know then you'll have to be more prepared in the event that you finally arrive on stage. The best part about this is that you make sure the person doesn't remember any details about the things they've performed while under the influence of hypnosis. Further details on post-show hypnotic memory in the future.

In your venue, select the music for your show carefully. Strange sounds, soaring synthesisers choruses and pulse-speed beats that will draw people into the kind of thinking you want them to. It is important to note that Kylie's "I'd Be So Lucky' does not convey the right vibe to it, regardless of the fact that it's your favorite track. It is not a good idea to think of luck being an aspect of your show. It's completely under your control.

If you have the money or if you have the ability, try your own music composed. The music you don't know will not cause any previously held thoughts in the mind of the audience. A well-known track like the work of Jean Michele Jarre's "Oxygene' might lead them to another place and you'd like to get to pay attention to them right now, here and now.

You now have your audience in the areas you'll need them. They've been flooded with expectations of entertainment and they ought to be aware of what they're expecting and many of them will even be eager to take the stage and be the star of your next show.

A few words here about safety at the site could be suitable.

You should do your best to ensure that dangers outside of your control are reduced to the greatest extent of your abilities. Speaker wires taped down. White marker tape placed one yard away off the front of stage. Seats are solid (rather as folding) when you are using seats that fold. Insurance for liability is paid. Accidents are not a good thing, so you should do everything to ensure your volunteers' safety. Your assistants are instructed to watch for anyone who is sitting on in the middle of the stage or on the stage. They are also excellent to keep an eye on the ones who aren't in a state of hypnosis, but only trying to ruin the show.

Think of everything you can do to cause trouble, and prepare for it or to mitigate it from happening or reduce the impact.

Hypnosis can be a bizarre thing. In several countries, if you use hypnosis to treat a patient, it is highly controlled, you require an approval, maybe accreditation and registration. However, stage hypnosis can be practiced anywhere, in the theatre, street or in a church, with no any restrictions in any way. And in other nations, like the UK for example it is completely reversed. Anyone can become a therapist, and there is less protest than an 'professional' organization (which may be a man working in his backroom office) who would like to be seen as regulating the field and wants an income, may be able to create. However, you should not stage a show using hypnosis without notifying the local authority 30 days prior to the show in order to apply for a permit, and you'll be in danger of being arrested in the event of a violation. In actual practice, no one has been detained for performing any kind of hypnosis-related show across the UK and to my knowledge, nobody was even stopped by a show that began. Even street hypnotists have hardly been asked to move forward.

My suggestion here is likely to be similar to what other professionals have to say. Examine the regulations of your country and, if applicable, state town, or county bye-laws because they can differ in accordance with the immediate locale. I've heard in certain countries, practicing with a friend who is willing to cooperate in your own home is not legal in the absence of a valid license which means you'll have be extremely cautious.

When it comes to practicing, it's obvious that you need to be consistent. While a lot of what happens when you start is dependent on the people you're working with, you need to be able to master your presentation to keep it moving and moving. Your opening remarks must be perfectly. If you don't do this, you won't be inspiring the audience by your capacity to manage. Your checklist must be jotted down as well as any audio and lighting signals you would like your technician to handle. If you require reminders, you can either create them in a very discreet manner and hidden from the public, so that they is unable to see them however you can reference them without being obvious, or conceal them from view - such as in a book that has a prominent striking black and yellow cover, labelled 'Hypnosis For Dummies to give yourself an additional laugh, though it may only work once or twice.

At first, practice with a small group of people and ask them to play with you' and pretend to be hypnotized. Ask one to play up as you progress. When you are able you can ask them to pick between them which one play with you at times and you're not sure what time or which. It's difficult to prepare yourself for scenarios where anything could occur however the more you ensure you are prepared for the worst, the more uncertain situations can frighten you. Now you have the advantage of having acquaintances who know your show and are your partner. They are aware of how they played your part and know what to watch out for if they see others trying to mimic your act in your performance.

Pilots of airlines must be trained every year twice in simulators for flight. In these simulation sessions, they will encounter more emergency situations in the space of four hours than they would in the course of flying in real aircraft. But if they've been taught to handle an engine fire during take-off, followed by complete electrical malfunction and wheels that refuse to lower, and a simple engine malfunction (reported to the public as a 'shocking air-related incident') is no more than a routine issue for pilots who've handled better, due to having trained repeatedly.

Do not settle for less regardless of the fact that nobody's lives are at risk and only your reputation is at stake. You are and should be ready for any situation.

One of the things that the modern stage hypnotist has to his (her) favor is the accessibility of video. Short clips or full-length shows that allow you to observe how other performers have achieved the same feat. You shouldn't duplicate everything exactly however, you can search for inspirations and concepts. Write a critique of the performance and try to identify areas in which the hypnotist could have handled things differently or in a better way. Keep in mind that you're benefiting from retrospective thinking and the ability to rewind or replay, something the performer was not able to do at the time.

One of the shows I was watching abruptly reduced the number of chairs to six. I returned to the show and saw that 4 of the performers weren't going back into trance as quickly as the other. When I watched the show from beginning to end I was able to see some indications earlier that two of the performers weren't as receptive as the others. They weren't intentionally resisting but they weren't willing to be a part of the group. Lessons learned, but not at my cost. One of them was to get rid of empty chairs. A chair that is empty shouts at the audience that you are not doing your job Therefore, get it removed quickly and as discretely as you can.

It's time to get the show started. Your announcer has called your name (Don't make it up yourself. The crowd will be able to hear your voice all night long) The hall lights are dimmed, the music is on, and your spotlight is waiting. This is happening now. The show is on!

## Chapter 13: The Fear of The Dark Thinking

Fear. The mere mention of it can cause an uneasy shiver through your spine. This is a reaction that we all share. The fear itself isn't a bad thing and I'd be the last person to wish to eliminate fear completely from someone however there are many areas of the human experience where fear can be detrimental.

Humans are fortunate to be in this situation. We're at the top in the chain of food should we choose we could be eating scorpions, sharks and lions... You can name it and be eating it. We can ignore the norms of society in this instance but there are ways in which we can improve our bodies with technology that allows us to be in the position of being in contact with predators that are alpha and still end up at the top.

In terms of evolution it is important to recognize the fact that fear led your to the place you're at here. It's an effective tool in terms of evolution. Because of our fear of darkness, for instance our ancestors may be more cautious in dark. The more enthusiastic members of the tribe might have ventured out into the dark only to be devoured by predators, thrown off a cliff into the darkness, tripped and fractured bones only to bleeding out, all this before they even had an opportunity to pass their genes onto the next generations.

What I'm trying say here is that we're naturally wired to be fearful of things. This is fine. Fear of darkness is a natural urge, but similar to the desire of children to pee when they have the desire it is possible to stop that urge. We can change our programming and work ways to overcome it. Don't be afraid of it. I've assisted hundreds of people like you feel more at ease in the dark, so let's do exactly the same thing for you now.

There's nothing to be worried about.

Do you find it like a calming sound? Perhaps, but let's try to determine the underlying cause that allows someone to remain in their current fearful state of mind when it comes to the dark. Children are taught that "there are nothing that you need to be scared of" and it sounds good to our rational, sensible conscious mind. However, it's not that part of our minds which is the source of the problem. It's our primitive, instinctual and (some may even claim) unconscious mind that is in charge of the endocrine system, it's the "fight or flight" response; the twitchy twisting, tingling and even gut-twisting incessant fear that's associated with fears, phobias and tiny quirks that make human beings such complex creatures.

In saying "there's no thing to be scared of" the thing we're actually doing is calling the darkness a thing. We label it "nothing" and claim it's something to be scared of.

Another way to say the same thing could be "there's something in the world. We refer to it as the "nothing," and you shouldn't need to be scared about it".

If you try to modify it, you'll face the same problem.

"Don't be scared. There's nothing to be afraid of. ..." to worry about." Wait... What? What's the Nothing? It's there! ?

Once you have named something, it acquires greater authority. The issue is that if you label something "nothing" The word "nothing" transforms into an adjective and begins to transform into something.

You're not messy, are you?

What are you able to do to solve this issue? I've been asked this question numerous times in my classes around the globe. The answer is pretty simple and comes in multiple components:

1.) Don't talk about it. Don't talk about the supposed nothing. If you make statements such as "there's nothing to worry about" or "nothing will harm you" You're (unwittingly) strengthening the anxiety.

2.) Say it. "But you've just declared that ..." that I'm sure of what I stated, and for majority of the time it's correct however, instead of simply relying on these terms the most important aspect is to clarify the root of your problems during the last time.

Did you know that I stated that the subconscious mind is extremely powerful? It's much more powerful over the mind of the conscious in lots of ways. It can take on greater amounts of input... The cognitive brain is also able to do something amazing when it comes to bringing about the necessary changes in your daily life. The most important one is providing insight into your subconscious mind.

Decartes stated "Cognito Ergo Sum" I am therefore I am. Humans are, to our limited knowledge, the only animal to possess of the ability to think and modify our own behavior using sophisticated critical faculties. We examine our own behaviors and motives, and possess the most extensive communication skills that we have to communicate the changes we would like to see happen in us as well as others. While the majority of animals (to in some way or in another) are able to modify their behavior to achieve their goals We don't see animals attending seminars or reading books about how to make changes.

Make use of this advantage. Utilize your mind's awareness to help you understand the problem. If you can see the things people say about their fear of the dark you'll realize that it's imprinted each time they speak things they're hoping to assist. It's not.

What can we do to help?

It is possible to begin thinking in a rational way and become aware of the definition of darkness. It is possible to explain how light functions. The concept of darkness is not real. It's not a bed or sheet or a massive cloud. It's not any of the things that novelists and poets insist it. This is just society reinforcing the an instinctual fear of its own goals. The poets and novelists would like people to believe in the notion that darkness is a reality. However, it's not. It's simply an absence of light.

Have a go with a trusted companion (or an intelligent home device If you're fortunate enough to possess one). Switch off the light for a moment. If you're unable to do that and many people are afraid to do so, because they have fears that stop them from doing it completely try turning it off with an dimming switch. If you're not comfortable delay, you can keep it on for a little longer than usual before turning on your home lights on. Let the sun's fading light reflect light onto your space. It's the same room, but it's different. There's nothing moving. The faces that you may observe when the light is gone aren't visible. They might only show up when the light is gone. Why is that?

The answer lies found in the biology of our species.

We form associations through the recognition of pattern patterns... Sometime even when the patterns aren't present! Psychologists refer to this phenomenon as paradolia. It makes complete sense. Think about it: far back in the past our ancestors took a walk for a stroll. They saw a face hidden in the bush. There are two possibilities that might be happening in this instance. It could be that there is faces or there's not. If there's no face anyone to care? Doesn't it? However, if there's... it's a good thing, because it could be friendly, or not. A sabre-toothed tiger may not be the best option to leap out of hiding behind the bush. If there were a danger it could result in the death of the individual and they would not be able to pass them to their children.

That's why the scared people who run; those who notice these forms and instantly go to safety in their homes, are able to survive. Does this mean there's nothing to be worried about for them. Not necessarily. Don't fast forward just a few million years into the present day. Similar neurological disorders occur within our heads, however the risks are greatly diminished and often completely illuminated. What's the chance of something lurking in the shadows of the living space? Perhaps in the sofa's shadow and ready to strike? Zero, right? You're aware of this but your brain is wired to a default state that's not the best for the modern world. Therefore, let's address that issue now through the hypnotic induced part of this program.

# Chapter 14: Classical Forms Of Suggestive Influence

Theories of the classical theorists of hypnosis

Suggestion as a method to influence the mind was well-known in earlier times, however because of the limitations of history of our human brains, it was unable to not be the subject of scientific study for years. However the religions have been used in various ways to influence the psyche. "God's shepherds" were only acquainted with the appearance of suggestion, but they also employed this psychological effect to establish their authority. One of the socio-psychological strategies that religions employ is suggestion.

The cults of various peoples and tribes throughout time have searched for methods which could be used to influence the human mind. Through this search for ways to use self-hypnosis, suggestion, and hypnosis and the transition of the psyche towards the state of twilight The yogis who have the greatest success.

Yogis provide a set of mental and physical exercise and exercises, which they claimed to help them achieve connection with supernatural forces. The early Egyptian writings "Vedas" the full explanation of the exercises that a yogi needs to complete to be able to control his body and the soul is offered. When in this state the yogi doesn't feel discomfort, and can be without food for a prolonged period of time, and without drinking water. If we do not believe in the religious component that is a part of the theories of Yogis, we must acknowledge that the technique of suggestion, autosuggestion , and hypnosis are extremely well-developed.

In 1530 around 1530, the Swiss doctor Paracelsus developed a theory according to which the health of humans depends on the effect of a particular magnetic fluid that is the electromagnetic radiation from celestial bodies.

Paracelsus (the known as Theophast Hohenheim) said: "There is one vital substance found in Nature that is the basis that is the basis of everything built. It's known as Archeus which means life force. It is associated to the light of astral, or an ancient spiritual air ... It is much lighter in substance than terrestrial body the ethereal body is more vulnerable to mismatches and impulses. The imbalance in this astral body is the reason for numerous illnesses. Someone with a troubled mind may poison his spirit and this disease can disrupt the natural circulation of the life force can later manifest as a physical condition ... ".

Over two centuries later, Viennese physician Franz Anton Mesmer created the theory and applied it according to its principles. Mesmerism's fundamental concepts are as below:

In order to be successful in treatment for mesmerists, they must be in good health;

The power of Mesmerich is contingent upon the specific features of the subject.

To attract, you must select a peaceful location that is easy to dress in. The process can also be affected by moral ambiguity, doubt;

The duration of the magnetic session increases between 10 and twenty minutes and then on.

Mesmer's most significant success was not in his pseudoscientific theories, but rather his method of immersion into trance and its connection to somnambulism. Mesmer realized that the therapeutic effects are superior in comparison to those who are in an euphoric state.

A significant step towards the development of a scientific explanation for the hypnosis phenomenon was taken in the time of Brad by Brad who published in the 1940s an article of hypnotism. Brad was then a French doctor, Nancy Liebo, who treated patients who had hypnotic ideas and also wrote a fascinating piece on this technique.

A significant part in the development of the subject is played by well-known neuropathologist Charcot who was a pioneer in the field of neuropathology, and demonstrated the Paris hospital hypnosis phenomenon to doctors who were hysterical around the globe. He believed that hypnosis was an abnormal nervous state that could be that is caused through physical mechanisms. But, Charcot met a sharp opposition to his ideas in the form of Professor Bernheim who caused an hypnotic state through the use of verbal suggestions and believed that hypnosis was an inspired dream, as well as the entire phenomena that occurs in hypnosis were due to the verbal stimulation alone. These differences played a significant role in the understanding of the phenomenon of hypnosis. This is the reason which is why the four researchers mentioned above should be considered to be the pioneers of the theory of hypnosis.

In denial of Sharko's view, Bekhterev says that most people are hypnotized at least some. It's not possible to acknowledge that everyone is hysterical. This idea was dealt the ultimate blow when it was realized that hypnosis must be acknowledged in animals to be a phenomenon which is totally similar and connected to the human experience of the process of hypnosis. If hypnosis, like we know it, is recognized in mammals, it's very natural that the source of its origins are in the world of organic life.

The study of suggestion in the psychophysiology and psychology in experimental research

Russian scientists shrewdly embraced the theory of magnetism in animals, but they also began to study the therapeutic and practical uses of mesmerists. Prof. at Kharkov University V.Ya. Danilevsky during a series of studies, examined hypnotic behavior in animals. He concluded in 1891 the state of hypnosis in humans and animals is alike in appearance. He described hypnosis as a state of paralysis and independence of thought, and thought that reason could be a form of mental coercion. However it was not the actuality.

The 4th Congress of the Society of Russian Doctors in Moscow in 1939, where V. Ya. Danilevsky delivered a report "On the therapeutic application of the hypnotism" The psychotherapist Ardalion Ardalionovich Tokarsky (1859-1901) gave an address. The entire speech and subsequent work of Tokarsky focused on an understanding of hypnosis from a scientific perspective. Tokarsky believed that the application of hypnosis is accessible to everyone however, it is possible to achieve success in this field be attained only by an in-depth understanding of the technique used to induce hypnosis and a thorough understanding of the phenomenon.

VM Bekhterev has been studying the specifics of the hypnotic state in man is able to conclude that hypnotic states play an important role when a verbal suggestion is made in addition to various physical stimuli which contribute to an individual's immersion into the state of hypnosis. He classified the hypnosis process into three phases - small medium, deep and small, which corresponded with the three commonly accepted stages of Trout hypotaxia, drowsiness and somnambulism. Bechterev was very interested in research that was aimed at identifying ways to enhance the effectiveness of suggestions given by a patient either during hypnosis or.

The foundation of the strategy of IM Sechenov-IP Pavlov lies in the principle of reflex. It is the basis of how the body develops (and sheds) its intravital functions in the form and structure of its behavior. From the viewpoint of nervism, the issues of resolving the activities of different departments of the brain as well as various levels of its organization including the molecular and neuronal level to the behavior of the entire organism are resolved, and the interplay between the processes of the brain's subcortical and cerebral cortex structures is examined. The method of teaching IM Pavlov on higher nerve activity developed by the influence of the traditional materialism of Russian philosophy, and he developed the concepts of IM Sechenov. The guiding was the idea of reflex self-regulation of the organism's work, which has an evolutionary-biological (adaptive) meaning. The primary role in self-regulation is carried out through the nerve system (the concept that neurism is the basis). In the beginning, he studied digestion and blood circulation, Pavlov went on to examine the behaviour of the whole organism, that is a unit of both internal and external manifestations as well as the relationship with the external surroundings. The organ that is responsible for this connection is the brain cerebral hemispheres' centers which are the highest integrator of all life-related processes, even the mental ones. This is a way of denying the dichotomy between physical and spiritual aspects.

## Chapter 15: Understanding Hypnosis

It is true that science appears to be in disagreement with a lot of this however, why is it that we continue to suffer from issues with our health, even with our supposedly modern science? In the past the human race had learned his mind as the strongest organ that could aid you in dealing with difficulties in life. This is the reason he learned to make use of hypnosis some of the difficulties which he encountered. Today it is utilized in the treatment of weight issues as well as self-esteem issues, ending addictions, curing depression , and many other issues that we all are struggling with. Understanding how to harness the potential of your mind can ensure that you have a happy and fulfilled life. How do you begin to adopt this ancient method to cope the challenges of life? Before we get into that, let me begin by introducing you to the basics of the nature of hypnosis and the various ways to use it.

What is Hypnosis?

Hypnosis refers to the induction of consciousness whereby a person loses the power of action through voluntary effort and becomes very attuned to any suggestion or direction. It is a state of trance which is generally marked by an extreme state of relaxation, enhanced imagination, and a high degree of possibility. It's not sleep, due to the fact that you're fully awake and alert when in an euphoric state. It's like daydreaming , or the sensation of being completely lost in a film or book in which you are completely aware, but you have shut off the noise which surrounds you. your attention is solely only on your subject and completely forget about all other thoughts.

Our brain, which is in its state of unconsciousness is not able to fully explore its potential. When we enter an hypnotic state it is possible to delve deeper into our minds and tune it to our desired thoughts to improve our thinking and behaviour.

It's the reason psychiatrists often employ hypnosis for psychological and mental problems due to its effectiveness in changing perceptions and behaviors.

Once you know the nature of hypnosis Let me assist you distinguish between the two main types of the hypnosis. Hypnosis can be classified into two broad categories, namely hypnosis and self-hypnosis.

If you require someone to help you enter the state that is known as a trance it is known as hypnosis. If you prefer to do all of it on your own, in your own way that is known as self-hypnosis. Each will result in similar outcomes. But, your choice between these two methods will be contingent on whether or not you're in a position to enter into a state of trance that's essential to the art of hypnosis. Naturally, the majority of us want to learn self-hypnosis in order to be sure that they are able to hypnotize themselves whenever they want , as rather than scheduling appointments with professionals which could be difficult and expensive. If you're among people who prefer to do things by themselves and are interested in learning more about self hypnosis, this book will guide you through the world of self-hypnosis that allows you to go into an euphoric state whenever you'd like, wherever. This will allow you to induce a state of hypnosis to gain one of the benefits listed below.

The Benefits Of Hypnosis

#To treat addictions

The majority of addictions are controlled by the mind and can be successfully managed with the aid of the power of hypnosis. Hypnosis is a great tool to overcome mental blocks which make it difficult to stop addiction. If you're looking to overcome any addiction then you should learn the skill of and self-hypnosis. It can help you avoid any return.

#For losing weight

The art of hypnotizing yourself can assist in the battle against cravings, by entering an euphoria or a state of numbness. You can also manage emotional issues, which could aid in the process of learning to manage emotional eating.

#To manage chronic pain

When diet or drugs fail to manage severe pain in cases of migraine, back pain, cancer pain, sickle cell disease pain, Temporomandibularpain, arthritis or fibromyalgia, you can incorporate hypnosis to help relieve pain.

#For reducing stress

Hypnosis can put the mind into the state of relaxation and assists in reducing stress or anxiety. When the mind has learned to manage its anxiety it also begins becoming more relaxed.

#To increase self-esteem

Our minds are the primary source of our personality-related troubles. Hypnosis assists in addressing these issues and increases confidence in ourselves. It trains our minds to avoid negative thoughts and to absorb the positive thoughts.

#For curing sleep disorders

If you've tried every medication available and every trick that you can think of to help you sleep then you should consider an approach to hypnosis that can help you deal with the issue. Since the majority of sleep disorders are psychologically-rooted in the mind, hypnosis can be effective in treating them.

#To improve behavior

Our behavior patterns are based on the type of childhood we experienced. If you are feeling that you are prone to aggressive, rude or angry behaviour, you could try hypnotizing yourself as attempt to address the issue. While your mind is at a deep level of hypnosis gets honed in order to rid it of negative beliefs and replace them with a positive perspective.

Once you know the effects of hypnosis Let me describe how it works to ensure you know how it functions when you're hypnotizing yourself. By understanding this, you will be certain of what you can be expecting from the experience to ensure that you don't end in a state of fear or disappointment.

How Hypnosis works

By using hypnosis, you or the hypnotist can communicate through the mind's subconscious. To learn deeper into how it happens I'm sure you are aware that the conscious portion of our brain is the one that we interact with each day In most cases it is possible to consider this part to be the person we are in reality but that's not the case. Your conscious brain is what is reading this article, while your subconscious is busy doing many other things , including performing different things that the conscious part of your mind isn't aware of.

To fully comprehend this your unconscious or subconscious mind is the one responsible for controlling all autonomic bodily processes like the generation of cells and blood pressure as well as heart rate, immune system and the growth of tissues, aging, and many more; it doesn't require you to think about them in order for these processes to take place. In addition the memories, experiences and thoughts are stored in this area of our brains. It is also responsible for regulating behaviors, emotions, and various other responses. For a deeper understanding Do you know that your subconscious mind manages around two million pieces of information every second, while the conscious mind is only able to control 7 bits? This means that only a small portion of what our subconscious mind processes gets into our conscious mind. It is as if our conscious mind is able to filter out the most important information and then leaves the remainder to the unconscious mind. In any event there is no processing capacity!

Your mind is analytical, critical and logical, which means it is required to evaluate situations through making judgements. Even if you're advised to quit smoking cigarettes since it's bad for your health, you will need to think about what you've been told, that is likely to cause you to question the advice. Whatever the situation, the conscious part of your brain is responsible for keeping your habits in place.

Your subconscious mind is quite open and tends to take things seriously and even literally particularly when it is related to your personal identity. The goal of hypnosis is to connect with your unconscious mind and bypass the conscious mind with relaxation or linguistic techniques, that allow you to talk directly to your unconscious mind using an understanding language which includes the language of metaphor, association, and patterns.

Although you may think that your mind's conscious is at the helm your subconscious mind is in control. Are you aware that certain actions that you've mastered to perform at the subconscious level are usually learned in a non-helpful way? For instance, smoking began as a joke because people thought that smoking was cool as an teen. After a few times, your unconscious mind is conditioned to the notion that smoking cigarettes is "good" and good for your health. Through hypnosis, the aim is to introduce valuable and fresh information into your mind's subconscious It is akin to the process to programming on a computer. By using this method you are able to input any information you want to, which can cause you to stop identifying any bad habit with pleasure, which means that you'll start looking at them from a completely different view of being poor, uncouth, or gross.

The purpose of hypnosis is to assign any habits or unwelcome feelings that you are experiencing to 1,999,993 bits of sensory data so that they do not become conscious because you're not conscious of any of them. You could describe it as a method of changing your view of real world by addressing your subconscious mind, which is where the majority of our problems originate and where the solution to these issues lie.

I am sure that you are amazed by the possibilities that the practice of hypnosis can bring. But, before you get into a state that is bliss where nothing else is important it is essential to create the perfect setting to relax in a state where you aren't distracted by any other thing. Hypnosis, also known as self-hypnosis is a technique that can be used in a relaxing environment that helps calm the mind and assist it stay clear of distractions. To practice self-hypnosis, the surroundings must be peaceful serene, peaceful and quiet. Learn how to make the perfect atmosphere for self-hypnosis. Before you can do that it is crucial to formulate auto-suggestions to help you navigate your self-hypnosis experience. We'll go over some guidelines for creating auto-suggestions and structuring them in our next section.

# Chapter 16: The Reasons Nlp is Working for Selp-Help?

It is believed that the Neuro Linguistic Program or the NLP can be a tremendous aid to individuals to build confidence in themselves and succeed in every endeavor. It's a fantastic training program that focuses on communicating, which is crucial throughout the day. Everyone is different from the individual in regards to attitudes, limits as well as skills and expertise. There are people who aren't able to show their self in public, and prefer to live a the most basic and boring life. In reality, if they decide to go through an NLP training, it might be possible to see how important the individual's relationship with his or her self.

Every person should be sure that they are in an open and clear communications with other people, perhaps with family and friends to be able to recognize the issues that they need to sort out and what they must eliminate. But, there are occasions where an individual isn't proficient in forming precise, concise and concise words to communicate, so they can't afford to shout their thoughts out. This is precisely the reason why NLP is effective and helps people build confidence in themselves. It's due to it being true that NLP training requires both human brain and ability in order to communicate effectively.

There are occasions where a person believes that he's very adept at communicating with others and believes that he will be able to use communication to elaborately explain himself. But when it's the time to make a statement it is as if all the words in his head or phrases he came up with before he started speaking disappear by the breeze. In this scenario the person will require NLP training. There are many types of NLP classes, so you must decide the one that suits you the best. You are the only person to decide which type of training you need to go to, since your are the sole person who understands your limits and abilities.

Two things you need to develop greatly are honesty and discipline. In addition, you need be able to think critically and objectively about what you are able to accomplish and attain in your communicating. Keep in mind that you'll require this if you wish to be successful with your NLP training and would like to take advantage of the benefits it will offer you with the ability to change your life to be a better person. People who are timid are not uncommon, however if they do not consider methods to overcome this, they could be putting themselves in a single spot or even worse, prison.

Jail implies that the person are unable to afford exploration and discover more about themselves because they are confined by their beliefs, which is exactly what is the purpose is behind "jail." If you realize that you're the type of person, then you must change your ways now and take part in NLP training as often as you can. It is a great way for people to discover and explore new aspects of themselves every day, by being able to communicate clearly and effectively to those in their lives. It's always pleasant to speak with a variety of people. Be aware that having a conversations with a variety of people could bring you closer to understanding and sharing experiences that could be a great way to learn or even gaining an understanding of who you are.

Many people say they know everything about their own personal information. However, the reality is that each person will continue to discover new aspects of themselves as long as they're acquiring new facts and realities. The possibilities are infinite, so you should think about the things you can accomplish, say, see and feel. When you are undergoing NLP training, you must make use of their senses, as it is crucial in the field of communication. Communication plays an important role in aiding you in achieving your goals.

Today, people need to be smart and improve their communication skills with other people. If you believe that you're not able to, then at the very least, you should begin communicating using chat, emails or emails. In the beginning, you will likely start writing your thoughts. In the future, you must consider having a discussion about it, perhaps with people you love initially, to become comfortable with it. In the end, you'll be able to see that you're halfway to your goal and that you're very proficient at communicating.

NLP is the reason for the success of every human being Neuro for your mind and linguistic to provide the highest quality communication that you require. This is crucial in helping yourself to achieve tangible and intangible goals. It is generally recommended that one think about NLP training, especially in the event that they would like to do whatever they want, but you're being restricted by your own self-limiting thinking and inadequate communication skills and lack of courage.

Making use of NLP to break down barriers...

NLP is a software program that is extremely beneficial for people who are struggling with their physical and mental communication abilities. It is a term used to describe Neuro Linguistic Programming which can open people's eyes on the significance of mental programming as well as an effective ways to communicate with others. Communication plays an important role in the development of every person, and this is among the reasons that explains the significance of NLP. It helps people communicate and help others understand them. Everyone wants to be heard and appreciated particularly if they were looking for something that's really difficult to attain, such as the job that requires strong communication ability.

However, NLP has also great capabilities when it comes to getting past mental obstacles. There are instances when people are afraid to speak or express themselves in a way that is their own. They prefer to let others criticize them and make decisions to them. Actually they could actually help them by being capable speak up for themselves. So, here are just a few of the ways where NLP can play a significant function in overcoming mental obstacles:

In the absence of courage, they did not succeed to achieve the goals they wanted to accomplish.

This is the reason for the greatest purpose of NLP in overcoming mental obstacles. It's fairly easy to explain the reason why people become shy about communicating with words, particularly when they need to speak to many people, or when they are required to give something to a specific individual. What's holding them back from speaking is their belief system and fear of being disregarded. NLP also explains that it's the fact that one is not always praised after speaking; and that's something to be acknowledged. Sometimes, one must experience rejections to examine his weaknesses. This will allow him to think of alternative ways to improve his self-improvement , so that the next time is when he will know exactly how to convey himself. In the majority of cases, after those rejections it is possible to develop more creativity and come up with important ideas that need to be expressed earlier.

Fear of making mistakes.

This is a fact that can be explained as there isn't anyone who would want to fail in their lives. If you focus at the bright side of life, you'll be able to see that a normal person requires a lot of failures in order to develop courage and determination to take on any challenge on their path. Neuro Linguistic Programming further explains the way that people be able to set up their minds so that they can achieve the things they desire. In addition they are able to precisely determine how they'll confront or deal with mistakes in a manner that is beneficial to them. So, they can overcome mental obstacles that hinder the confidence and determination to step out into the world they've always wanted to be.

It can cause people to come out of their shells and raise their chins raised.

A majority of people fail when they had to stand up for their own self in front of many people, because they feel too ashamed to do it. NLP will greatly assist individuals to get from their shells with their chins raised. This means they are able to face the crowds and also communicate freely without limitations, neither emotionally, nor mentally. This is why people have a difficult to speak for themselves, as they might have experienced previous events which make them hesitate. This is the reason why NLP could be of huge aid to people as it allows people to slowly overcome their doubts and fears.

If you think you're facing these issues within yourself, then think about getting NLP training or at least conduct an extensive search to find out the training and program is about. In this way, you will be able to learn about its fundamentals in your own scenario you'd like. In the end, learning about different facts independently could be beneficial, especially since trainings and participation are costly these days.

But, this doesn't mean to suggest that you shouldn't invest some money in developing the concepts or the teachings of NLP. Of sure, there are situations which you need to. The main thing is that you must find instances that help you reduce costs when studying it. If you can you'll need courage as well as skill and experience in order to master things on your own. If you believe that you possess these, then you can accomplish almost anything you've always wanted to do in your life.

It's all it takes, and you'll need to determine if you'll require NLP training or if you are able to take it on your own. Keep in mind that if you are looking for a precise assessment , you have to make it up to your self as nobody else is able to determine the results on your behalf, but you yourself.

## Chapter 17: Redefining The Mind

There are two options in this case. We can alter the mental state or alter our the chemistry of our body. Does that sound complicated? It's not.

For the mind there is no distinction between the actual state and the one that is constructed. You are well aware of this in fact, as you employ it often to help you demotivate yourself. It's true. You must be motivated. Think about your last experience when you been a failure, and you'll feel more relaxed even if it was 20 years ago. Imagine your girl(boy)friend sleeping with a different person and you'll feel insecure and angry. What's going on? It didn't even happened! For the mind, there is no difference between real Experience and Imaginary.

What can we do? Imagine ourselves feeling Well.

The second method of changing your mental state is to change the chemistry of your body. It's not easy. It's not. The secret is that our body's chemical composition is dependent on our physiology. To simplify, anything you do with your bodies will impact the body's chemistry. If you overdo your physical exercises, you'll experience sore muscles. This is because there is a build-up of the lactic acid inside the muscles. It's a chemistry in your body.

How can you be content? You smile. It's a shift in your physiology and it can alter the chemistry of your body and will alter the state of your mind. It's a simple answer after all that research!

What happens If you combine these two methods? Sit straight and unwrap your shoulders. breathe deeply (breathing can be the most effective method to alter the body's chemical balance. It eliminates $CO_2$ from the bloodstream, and gives you oxygen, altering the blood's pH... And it makes you feel good, particularly when you haven't done it in the last 30 minutes or longer) And now, make sure you smile on your face. It's not your typical "light as well as relaxed" smile that they inform you in one of the "quit smoking cigarettes in just 21 minutes for $129.99 with tax" lessons however, a huge smile. Yes, I'm inviting you to see whether you can smile like a DUMMY. Of course you do as you read this book. If you believe there's no reason to be happy, take a look at yourself in the mirror and smile at the dummy because you deserve it. Does he not look funny with that smile?

Then the magic takes place. In just 30- 60 second, your body's physiology will alter your mind's state of mind. It will completely erase any previously existed state. Your state of mind will change. You can now read the book and keep smiling. The book is great and, if you're lucky, it may alter your life. The smile can change your life and luck does not have anything to do with it.

Stories of success.

My approach was more than simply describing the advantages of smiling to you , but convincing you to smile. It's time to smile... just like every time when someone is trying to convince you to take action... You're faced with an option. You have the option of doing it or do something different. It is crucial to note, though it is not always explicit in NLP books to understand that NLP is about making the right choice for yourself , whereas the actual techniques are methods. The philosophy starts with.

There are several presuppositions that are referred to as Presuppositions of NLP (unfortunately at present SMLIE isn't one of them. The presupposition is part from The Introduction to State of Power). The main distinction between NLP and the majority of others "teach you how to train your self how to succeed" techniques is in the way that it teaches these presuppositions to you. It's not the ultimate truth, NLP says. When you consider it, it's not even a reality. It's nothing more than a an assortment of Convenient beliefs. It is your choice to accept the beliefs.

What will these beliefs do to you? They'll alter how you view the notion of success, as well as your personal capabilities. One example is that one of the assumptions is that "what one person is able to accomplish, another man can learn, too". Wait a minute! It basically implies that I am able to do almost anything! Do I have to believe it?

Since this is what they'd say in other theories of thought trying to get your attention, here's John who hails from Wyoming. He was an (looser and drunk, unemployed, can think of it) prior to his decision to work in NLP (it is expensive staff, so where did this drunk obtain this cash?). Three months later, the president is now a part of a successful business and father of three kids (three children in just three months! We're telling you, THIS PERSON IS POWERFUL! )...

The thing is, it's the success story. I'll admit it, they can do it in NLP as well. However, let's get rid of the nonsense, because in the end, this book is meant for people who are able to use a critical eye and smile when doing it. It's true that is if you take an average human being and ask him or them to do anything... it is likely that the changes will usually be positive. All you have to do is let this coach go and make a change. Get more vegetables. Reduce your intake of vegetables. Exercise. Avoid wasting energy. Take part in classes for motivation. Beware of those psychos who teach their classes. Any new thing is beneficial for you, and... it's at the very least, it's more beneficial than nothing at all.

Yes, we could locate John from Wyoming who did this and achieved success. And if it's not so, we could always create a new story. That's not the issue.

If we practice something for repeatedly enough, we begin to become proficient at it. As we get betterat it, our behavior is automatic. When you ask a toddler when it is but nothing will happen. If you ask me, my left hand will shift in a slight manner, even though I am not wearing a watch in the moment. A habit.

It's the same in thinking about success as well as failure. Let's consider something. Imagine, you are approaching an attractive woman (if you're a male. In order to make room in this book I usually call someone "he" instead of "she" simply because I'm a male Men are lazy, as well "she" is an additional character rather than "he") as well prior to engaging with a woman, you are thinking of every possible way to be unsuccessful, what would occur? It is likely that you will not succeed. Maybe you wouldn't attempt to meet her. It is extremely scary knowing that you'll be a failure. Isn't that right?

This is what success stories are for. You learn stories about John of Wyoming and then you imagine yourself in his shoes. It's nice to imagine yourself as an award-winning person, doesn't it? Three months later, he was blessed with three kids? I now have five children and I'm looking for the chance to eliminate two suckers? Hey, here's my card! Is my wife eligible? Can I... Just kidding...

## Chapter 18: What Hypnosis Can and Can't Do

"The Webster's New International Dictionary defines the term hypnosis as "the inducement of a state that resembles sleep or somnambulism that is referred to as hypnosis or hypnotic sleeping; or, more loosely, the state of induced of the hypnotic state."

There are various degrees of hypnosis that have been described as "lethargic cataleptic, somnambulistic, and lethargic hypnosis." Another is simply as heavy and light somnambulistic sleep, with the similar variations in the degree of hypnosis."

However in Encyclopedia Britannica also states that "there is no universally accepted explanation for hypnosis. However, one popular theory is based around the potential of dissociative discrete states that alter certain aspects of the mind."

The word "hypnosis" comes of the Greek word hypnos, which means sleep. It is believed that hypnosis can cause a person to enter an altered state of consciousness, even though the person is awake. The typical behavior of people in hypnosis is that the subjects are highly responsive to suggestions, and attain an extremely relaxed state. Daydreaming is a different activity that can be compared to hypnosis, where one is completely unaware of the world around him but experiences an increased imagination (depending on the depth of the trance).

There are two methods by the hypnosis process is carried out: (1) hetero-hypnosis, where a hypnotist causes an experience of trance, and is open to suggestions, or (2) auto-hypnosis, in which the state is created by self-induction. This latter type of hypnosis is also known as self-hypnosis. In fact it is all selfhypnosis since no hypnotist is able to create hypnosis without the person's consent. The same results can be expected whether it is done by a hypnotist or oneself, however some people are more likely to enter hypnosis in the presence of an professional hypnotist.

A suggestion that occurs over for a time period following the hypnosis process is called post-hypnotic suggestions.

It's true that we are hypnotized every day. Are you so lost in an audiobook or a film that you didn't hear that someone was calling you at the high pitch? Did you miss an exit driving on the highway due to the fact that you were absorbed in your thoughts? Have you ever been caught thinking about your daydreams in class instead of paying attention to your teacher? Writing, reading or hearing music can be just a few instances of activities that induce a state of mind, thereby altering our focus so that we are highly attentive and unaware of off other subjects that are competing at our attention. Anything that is intensely focused on your attention is an act of hypnosis.

In addition, we can be too absorbed by the fictive world of a dream or an entire chapter in the book that our emotions are triggered. We cry over a emotional song, or feel terror when the villain approaches the protagonist's place of refuge in a book or scream in the face of the most frightening scenes. Many churches also employ the principles of hypnosis during their repeated sermons. Have you heard of "religious passion?"

This type of thing known as self-hypnosis is so frequent and is a common feature which Milton Erickson, a hypnosis specialist during the 20th century, and often referred as the founder of modern hypnotherapy, found that people are hypnotized every day. Hypnosis can be called "controlled dreaming."

Be aware that this type of "everyday trance" is distinct from the trance that is induced through deep hypnosis and is similar to the relaxed state of mind that occurs between the hours of the state of sleep and wakefulness. Also, there is a distinction between auto-hypnosis where the state of extreme suggestion is self-induced, and hetero-hypnosis, in which it is brought on by a hypnotist or a different person. We will attempt to further explain in the subsequent chapters.

In all the previously described categories, the person who is hypnotized according to Encyclopedia Britannica, "seems to respond in a noncritical manner, and automatic, while disregarding aspects of the surroundings (e.g. sounds, sights) not mentioned by the expert hypnotist. The subject's memory and perception of themselves may change due to suggestions and the effects of suggestions can be carried over (post-hypnotically) throughout the person's subsequent activities in the waking world. ...."

In self-inducing hypnosis the person is relaxed and extremely open. Any worries regarding reality "real world" are deemed to disappear briefly while reading an ebook or in a movie.

It is similar to the hypnosis process using the professional hypnotist. If the hypnotist says that the subject is experiencing intense heat, that subject could begin sweating and suffer from high temperatures even if the temperature is pleasant. If he tells an insecure and hesitant person that he's an extremely confident and confident man who is confident of himself, the individual may suddenly feel more comfortable with others, even strangers.

A seasoned and knowledgeable hypnotist is the one to acknowledge that the effects will occur for the duration of time, unless person really wants to make a change. For instance, a person is hypnotized to stop smoking by convincing them that smoking cigarettes is harmful and dangerous. This person may then be afflicted by smoking and feels nauseated every time he is near it. Thus, he may shun cigarettes. However, if the individual doesn't want to quit smoking or if they is smoking for someone other than themselves The habit will be brought back in time.

Another limitation to the practice of hypnosis is that basic beliefs, common sense of belief, convictions and beliefs remain in place throughout and following the experience. It is impossible for anyone to be hypnotized at will since the mind needs to be willing and open to being influenced by the hypnotist's ideas.

For instance, hypnosis can't cause the Muslim consume pork or make an Superman fan fly through the window. The mind is completely alert (only your subconscious remains alert) the person's senses of security are constantly on guard. His senses will continue guide his decision-making process. However we will never be certain. A story tells of one man who was under the hypnosis process to boost his confidence and was advised by the hypnotist the man "could accomplish anything, any thing provided he puts his thoughts into it." To further enhance the impact, the hypnotist claims: "Why, you could even steal a bank if wish to." Though the hypnotist could have meant this as an example, the subject does indeed take a bank hostage in the next few days! There are two things to worth noting: one the hypnotist was indecent when he made such a suggestion, even if it was meant as an illustration, and, secondly taking the action of robbing banks was already a part of the subject's basic values. Or put in other way, the person's moral compass wasn't functioning at all. Hypnosis can't force you to perform a task that you wouldn't normally perform.

A study has revealed that in the average, 25 of 100 people are easily hypnotized. Most children are in this category, and are thought to be very vulnerable to suggestions. The proportion of this is dependent on the hypnotist's personality, style and expertise. The effectiveness of the expert hypnotist is also dependent on the person's personality and attention span as well as mental state at the time. It is interesting to note that while it appears reasonable that those with exceptional intellects aren't able to be attracted by hypnosis due to their ability to process every piece of information that enters their brains, it's in reality the reverse. The belief is that people with intelligence tend to be the best creative. Therefore, they are able to easily connect the hypnotist's words with their own sensory or visual representations. People with strong analytical skills that are the hardest to manipulate since they can't stop looking at what the person who is hypnotizing them.

It's commonplace to hear people say "I cannot be hypnotized" and they're right. If you believe that you can or can't be hypnotized you're right. It's all up to you.

Warnings and words of Caution

Hypnosis is an impartial force that is neither good nor harmful. Its effectiveness is contingent on the person the person who uses it and how it is utilized. Mind control, also known as the power of suggestion, as well as accessing the unconscious is a risk if used in a reckless manner. But, hypnosis is not able to be used to manipulate others, however brainwashing could be used to control others if carried out over a long amount of time. Examples of brainwashing include intelligence agents and followers of religious cults.

Hypnosis can also be associated with creating false memories. Therefore when doing research like abductions from aliens or past-life regressions or similar cases, it is not recommended that hypnotists introduce information in the hypnosis session that the subject hasn't previously stated or offered. It is similar to "leading to the person" and may result in concocting outcomes. Confabulation refers to the process of putting false memories on an individual to fill in gaps in memory. It is a no-no when it comes to the art of hypnosis.

Hypnosis is more susceptible to abuse since it does not require much effort to understand how to use it. Anyone can learn to practice it and attain a certain amount of success. Although the effects could be short-term or even minimal but hypnosis does have the ability to change some aspect of how the person is able to think about, behave, or even decide for the future.

In this context, caution should be exercised when working with the practice of hypnosis. In the first place regardless of whether it is handled by a trained professional it isn't a panacea on its own. It's most effective when it is utilized in the right proper method, and when used in conjunction with other therapies that are similar. It's not a substitute for medical or psychotherapy.

So, only a trained person can attempt to identify the person, and determine the factors that affect the individual; and then recommend a suitable treatment. The doctor will be able provide an accurate evaluation of the particular case.

In contrast, a non-trained person may misdiagnose the condition and arrive at an inaccurate or incorrect diagnosis and recommend the wrong treatment.

It is recommended to seek advice from a medical professional instead of hypnosis when a person is suffering from an illness or pain. Doing so may cause life-threatening complications. Pain is the body's method to tell us there is something wrong. Imagine if you could hypnotize the pain of someone with a serious health issue. In the event that the patient you had hypnotized didn't not experience the pain caused by the illness, they would not see a doctor for a health check-up. This could result in potentially unsafe outcomes, and could negatively impact the health and lifestyle of the person.

Be aware when you use the hypnosis method. When you have power, comes accountability.

# Conclusion

Hypnosis is a constant aspect of our lives whether we've realized it , or not. It's because the capability to listen and respond to non-verbal or spoken suggestions, without conscious analysis or evaluation is an integral aspect that makes us human. It's that simple.

Our capacity to absorb our attentionand investigate and change the connections that have formed in our mental'map of the universe' these are also fundamental to being human.

Hypnotism can be described as not just an art, but it is also a technique, even though it's not a requirement that we must master or acquire. This is perhaps the most amazing aspect of hypnosis for me. MP3s. We can instantly access the expertise and talents of any hypnotherapist we preference from the top around with us at any time and for a price that is unbelievable and all we have to do is shut our eyes, take a deep breath and take in the experience.

www.ingramcontent.com/pod-product-compliance
Lightning Source LLC
Chambersburg PA
CBHW071838080526
44589CB00012B/1036